"During my peak ultrarunning years, I started to see the long hours on the trail as a practice of something deeper than solely logging miles. Running became my vehicle to explore the connection between body and mind, and ultimately a deeper sense of my being. In *Still Running*, Vanessa Zuisei Goddard vividly guides us on a journey of moving into stillness, escorting us on a path of transferring those road and trail miles to our daily lives."

—SCOTT JUREK
ultramarathon champion, *New York Times* bestselling author of *North* and *Eat and Run*

"This is a lovely and unusual book, a book that speaks about the spiritual and meditative aspects of running. I enjoyed reading this book, which contains engaging mindfulness practices that can be applied not just to running but to seated meditation and many other activities in life. These practices will help the reader develop the most important aspect of spiritual practice, deep inner stillness, which becomes a reliable source of stability and ease in all aspects of life. The writing is fresh, succinct, inspiring, and laced with insights from the author's three decades of running and two decades of intensive Zen practice."

—JAN CHOZEN BAYS
author of *Mindful Eating* and *Mindfulness on the Go*

STILL

RUNNING

The Art
of Meditation
in Motion

Vanessa Zuisei Goddard

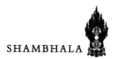

SHAMBHALA

Shambhala Publications, Inc.
4720 Walnut Street
Boulder, Colorado 80301
www.shambhala.com

© 2020 by Vanessa Zuisei Goddard

Cover art: Ashley Seil Smith
Cover design: Daniel Urban-Brown
Interior design: Kate Huber-Parker

9 8 7 6 5 4 3 2 1

First Edition
Printed in the United States of America

♾ This edition is printed on acid-free paper that meets the
American National Standards Institute Z39.48 Standard.
♻ Shambhala Publications makes every effort to print on recycled paper.
For more information please visit www.shambhala.com.

Shambhala Publications is distributed worldwide by
Penguin Random House, Inc., and its subsidiaries.

Library of Congress Cataloging-in-Publication Data
Names: Goddard, Vanessa Zuisei, author.
Title: Still running: the art of meditation in motion /
Vanessa Zuisei Goddard.
Description: First edition. | Boulder: Shambhala, 2020. |
Includes bibliographical references.
Identifiers: LCCN 2019035427 | ISBN 9781611808193 (paperback)
Subjects: LCSH: Meditation—Zen Buddhism. |
Running—Religious aspects—Buddhism.
Classification: LCC BQ9288 .G63 2020 | DDC 294.3/4435—dc23
LC record available at https://lccn.loc.gov/2019035427

To my father,
Eduardo Goddard,

who loves me and lives straightforwardly,

and for my teacher,
Geoffrey Shugen Arnold Roshi,

who embodies the dharma so thoroughly.

For one who clings, motion exists; but for one who clings not, there is no motion. Where no motion is, there is stillness. Where stillness is, there is no craving. Where no craving is, there is neither coming nor going. Where no coming nor going is, there is neither arising nor passing away. Where neither arising nor passing away is, there is neither this world nor a world beyond, nor a state between. This, verily, is the end of suffering.

—The Buddha,
Udana Sutta

Contents

Introduction

If you let go a little, you will have a little peace.
If you let go a lot, you will have a lot of peace.
If you let go completely, you will be free.

—Ajahn Chah

"If you find a book you really want to read but it hasn't been written yet, then you must write it," the novelist and Nobel laureate Toni Morrison once said.

When I decided to write a book about running and meditation, I knew it would have to be about more than these two disciplines. In order to say what I wanted to say, it would have to be a book about freedom, ease, and the joy of movement. It would be about mind and body and their interrelatedness. It would speak about the power of stillness and silence and the ways in which we can use that power in our lives.

My premise is simple. I believe it's more fulfilling to live life awake than asleep. I mean "awake" in both a practical and spiritual sense. We are awake when we remain present within each moment, responding skillfully to what is in front of us. Awakening is also enlightenment or liberation—the realization of who we truly are and what reality is made of. In the 2,500-year-old tradition of Buddhism, the main path to liberation is meditation, or as it's called in Zen, *zazen*, seated meditation.

My first Zen teacher, Daido Roshi, used to say, "Zazen is not contemplation, it's not meditation, it's not concentration. It's not quieting the mind or focusing the mind. Zazen is a way of using your mind. It's a way of living your life and doing so with other people." He meant that zazen is not about being quiet. It's not just about focusing or even about gaining insight on the meditation cushion. Zazen must function in our everyday lives, for if it's not working there, it's not really working.

I myself have been practicing this form of seated meditation for more than two decades, and I can attest to its power. At the same time, I've seen that, by itself, zazen will not necessarily lead to an awakened life. For, as difficult as sitting still and quiet for long hours can be, it's nothing compared to the challenge of taking that same stillness, concentration, and insight and applying it to everything that we do: the way we work, raise our families, or form relationships with one another. That's why we must learn to make the transition between stillness and movement, being and doing.

First we need to learn to *move into stillness* to make contact with our basic clarity and wisdom. Then, from that stillness, we must *move out into activity*, letting that clarity inform the way we live day to day. This is the functioning of compassion. And while I wouldn't claim that jogging a few miles a day will lead to enlightenment or compassion, I do see running meditation as an excellent entry point into the deep exploration of the nature of body and mind *within* daily life. Running zazen—which I call *still running*—can show us that fundamentally there is no difference between stillness and movement, body and mind, self and other. And this, the Buddha said, is the realization that leads to the end of suffering.

Finding My Way to Zen

My own journey to Zen Buddhism began years ago during a sort of pilgrimage. While in college I decided to take some time off and spent a couple of months backpacking through Europe. I needed time alone to reflect on what I was doing with my life and also to find a way to address the conflict I was seeing both in myself and in the world around me. Everywhere I went, I saw people of all ages and backgrounds struggling to get and keep things, struggling to form and maintain relationships, struggling to find meaningful and lasting forms of enjoyment. I would think to myself, *Is this it? Is this the only way to live a human life?*

One day, looking for a pen at the hostel where I was staying, I found in the drawer of the bedside table a book on Zen. Curious, I picked it up and began reading, not knowing that this simple act would change my life. (I have since wondered what would have happened if that drawer had contained a Bible instead.) While I had vaguely heard about zazen, I wasn't particularly interested in doing it—until that moment. As soon as I began following the meditation instructions delineated in the book, I was hooked.

At the time I knew almost nothing about Buddhism, and I had little context for the practice of zazen. Yet I felt compelled to meditate in a way that I couldn't have explained even to myself. I was used to getting up early to run, so now I woke up even earlier to sit quietly and count my breath. Although I had no idea what I was doing and couldn't tell whether zazen was even working for me, getting up every morning to sit like this felt like the sanest thing I'd ever done.

After about six months of practicing zazen on my own I began to feel I needed more guidance, so I did some research and found Zen Mountain Monastery a few hours away, in upstate New York. Excitedly, I signed up for an introductory weekend, and a few days later I took the bus up from Philadelphia. The driver dropped me off just outside the monastery gate, and as I walked through it, I heard a voice inside me say, "I'm home."

I loved everything about the weekend. I loved the stillness, the silence, the simplicity, and discipline of Zen. I signed up for another retreat, then decided to apply for a monthlong residency. Two days after graduation I moved into the monastery. My month there turned into a year, and at some point I realized I had found my calling. I could sense even then that zazen was the most powerful tool I'd ever encountered to study my mind. And the more I learned about Buddhism, the more it seemed to me that it was addressing the root of human conflict—the fundamental problem I'd grappled with during my travels, and which I eventually distilled into a single question: why does life have to be so hard?

For the next twenty years, I spent my days doing zazen, working, and studying. Besides the traditional reading of Buddhist texts, the residents were required to do *art practice* and *body practice*—creative expression and movement or exercise—as means to study the self. Because I had grown up playing sports, body practice especially appealed to me.

I learned that, unlike religious traditions that deny the body or see it as an obstacle to union with the divine, Buddhism offers that our physical being is the vehicle of our awakening. Because it is indivisible from mind, the body is the means through which we realize our interconnectedness with all things—our "interbeing," as the Vietnamese Zen teacher Thich Nhat Hanh calls it. So whether we were doing yoga, *qigong*, or *taiji*, we were meant to engage each of these forms of body practice as *moving zazen*.

After participating in these sessions for many years and eventually leading them, I realized that I could apply this same intent and awareness to running, the form of movement I know and love best.

Running as Self-Study

Running has been my main form of exercise for the past thirty-five years. I began running when I was ten years old, and over the years my reasons for doing it have changed as I've changed. I've run for exercise, comfort, escape, and glory. I've run out of fear, out of joy, and out of my need to identify myself as a runner and an athlete. Most often I've loved it, but on occasion I've resented it to the point of loathing. I've been asleep to it and suffered the consequences. I've been awake within it and felt the wonder of a moving, healthy body. On rare occasions, I've even felt myself disappear into movement. But the more I run, the more I see the immense potential this art has to teach us about the fundamental nature of the self.

Let me clarify, however, that the teachings I offer here are not limited to running. Walking, swimming, and bicycling are also excellent forms of moving zazen because of their repetitive, meditative nature. Even if you use a wheelchair, you can apply the same principles of concentration, mindfulness, working with the body, and working with the mind to your own form of body practice. Less important than the kind of movement you do is the *way* you use your body and mind. One of the main reasons I chose running as my focus is that it's accessible. All you need is a pair of running shoes, relatively good health, and willingness. In my running workshops, I've taught people of all abilities and ages (the oldest was almost eighty). So if you're wondering whether still running is for you, just remember what Reverend Martin Luther King, Jr., once said: "If you can't fly, run; if you can't run, walk; if you can't walk, crawl; but by all means keep moving."

There's no question that as a form of exercise running can help to keep your mind fresh, your body healthy. But with a bit more effort it can also teach you something about who you are.

Finally, a word of explanation about the language in this book. On occasion, when quoting from texts that were traditionally and exclusively male-centered, I've changed male pronouns to female in order to be more inclusive. More rarely, in my own examples I've opted to use the increasingly accepted epicene singular "they." In both cases, I believe these changes do not affect the substance of the material.

In addition, the language I use to describe running as a spiritual practice reflects the many years I've spent steeped in Buddhism, but you don't have to be a Buddhist—or a runner, for that matter—to benefit from reading this book. The only thing you need is to be interested in yourself and in the ways your understanding of that self affect the world you live in. Maybe you picked up this book because you've been wanting to develop a meditation practice and a Buddhist approach appeals to you. Maybe you can claim years of running experience and now feel ready to explore

STILL RUNNING

1

Practice

It is the kind of day that makes your feet feel like they're melting into the pavement, that makes the roof of your mouth hurt at the thought of ice cubes. Summer hasn't even had a chance to settle in, so the afternoon has no business being this hot. Yet here it is, and here we are—a few dusty, tired, but loyal friends and the track-and-field coaches, all wishing we could be somewhere else, be someone else. Anything to avoid this infernal heat.

We are standing on the sidelines of my high school's beat-up clay track, waiting for the 5,000-meter race. Normally I would have packed my gear and gone home long before, but my friend Juan is running, and I've promised to cheer him on. Just a couple of weeks earlier he'd been a swimmer, and a good one. But he'd earned his nickname—Colt—when he showed that his skill in the water paled in comparison to his speed on land. During our last cross-country race, he'd been so far ahead of the pack that, before he even crossed the finish line, our coach ran over to have a chat with the head of the swimming team. Now Colt is one of us.

I take a long swig from my water bottle and look to where Colt is standing, just behind the starting line. He is jumping lightly up and down on the balls of his feet and shaking out his long, slender arms in time with the other runners. But unlike them, he looks perfectly at ease, as if he's run hundreds of races (it is his first track race). Even the heat doesn't seem to bother him. He looks relaxed and poised, while the other runners keep fidgeting with their shoelaces, the drawstrings of their shorts, the numbers on their shirts. I feel a little sorry for them.

The starter gives the signal for everyone to get into position, and when the pistol goes off the men lunge forward as one body. For a few laps, four of them—including Colt—are shoulder to shoulder and slightly ahead of the rest. When one of them surges briefly, he is quickly reeled in by the others. Then someone else digs in, and again the others rush to catch up. So it goes for a while, a mass of legs and arms swinging, cleats pounding on dry clay, while the rest of us swelter on the sidelines.

Gradually, Colt begins to pull ahead. The others try hard to rein him in, but by the seventh lap he's had enough of their crowding, and suddenly he opens up his stride and pushes hard to get clear of the group. By the ninth lap, he has a comfortable lead and looks like he is thoroughly enjoying himself. He runs easily, his strides long and graceful and light, his face open. At one point he looks like he isn't even *there*. There is just running. Pure movement, pure action without agent, without goal, without time.

If I could only live my life as he runs, I think, *it would be a life well lived.* I don't even know what I mean exactly, but watching Colt run, I feel something in me shift. I understand that what I'm witnessing goes beyond the act of running, but also that it is not particular to my friend, although he embodies it so beautifully. His running is both *all* him and not him at all.

Colt keeps running easily all the way to the end, snapping the tape with a 300-meter lead while our small crowd cheers wildly. I rush forward to congratulate him, wanting to tell him what I've just seen. But something in his stance stops me. He looks happy in a basic, almost childish way, and I sense that speaking about his running would shatter the moment. So I keep my insight to myself, but I never forget it. I can sense that underneath Colt's utter unselfconsciousness lies the possibility of true freedom. And

I decide right then that if there is a path, a method to achieve this level of ease, I will find it. Even if I have to dedicate the rest of my life to it.

Running as Practice

To practice means to perform an activity or skill repeatedly in order to improve our proficiency in it. *Spiritual* practice is the constant and deliberate turning of our attention toward the fundamental questions of a human life. Who am I? What is life? What is death? What is reality? What is truth? In Buddhism, these questions are addressed primarily through the practice of zazen. But we can also apply this concept of practice to other areas of our lives. To practice an activity means to do it with focused attention and a deep desire to be awake to and within it. It's a desire to understand what is happening, not just on the surface of things but at a fundamental level—the level of ultimate reality. So to be awake means to see that reality clearly. It means not taking our thoughts, our ideas, our beliefs, or our actions for granted. Not assuming that we know and understand what we haven't carefully studied and deeply pondered.

For example, as I write these words, I can hear the steady tapping of my fingers on the keyboard. I could explain this sound as longitudinal waves moving through the air and reaching my ears. But if I were to put on noise-canceling headphones, what would happen to the sound? As the age-old question asks, does the sound exist if no one hears it? Is the sound in the keys, in my ears, in my mind?

Zen is not abstract. It is the study of reality for the sake of living that reality wisely and compassionately. But to do this we must first see things, not as we would like them to be, not as we think they should be, but as they really are. So in this context, practice is also the repeated effort of letting go of the thoughts, assumptions, and distractions that prevent us from seeing clearly. *Body practice* is the practice of using body and mind in order to clearly understand that very body and mind.

Ultimately, practice is no different from life. Each one of us goes through our days doing all sorts of ordinary activities: working, eating, walking, sleeping. Practicing these means engaging them with undivided attention—it means to "do what we're doing while we're doing it," as one of my teachers used to say—in order to see the nature of both action and doer.

Many runners run automatically. Many runners want to have finished running, but prefer to not be there while it's happening. Both of these do a disservice to the runner and to running. I'd like to show that being present is much more fulfilling, enjoyable, and worthwhile. This is what the practices at the end of each chapter are meant to do.

The mantras, visualizations, and other practices I've designed over the years are meant to help runners develop awareness of themselves, not just as physical beings, but also as emotional and spiritual creatures. To me, this is an essential component of awakening: to gain access to the full range of our being so that we can live in harmony with ourselves and with one another. These practices are also meant to bring us into closer contact with the act of running itself, to help us run safely and effortlessly.

I call them "practices" rather than exercises for three reasons: one, to stress the deliberate turning of our attention toward our bodies, our minds, and the act of running. Two, to move away from the limited definition of running as fitness training. When we see running solely as exercise, focusing on calories lost, pounds shed, and miles covered, we miss the deeper implications of this art. And three, to point out that running—like any other discipline— is an activity that each of us must choose to continue over time. Each day we have to choose to run with the understanding that, as a practice, running needs to change as we change. We're evolving human beings, not machines, which means our desires shift or fade over time. What we thought was important at one point in our lives doesn't seem so pressing at another. So don't be discouraged if you go through periods when you just don't want to run. It happens to everyone. Maybe you no longer get out of running what you originally did. Maybe other things in your life have taken priority. Maybe you've gotten older, and running the same way you used to is no longer possible.

It takes clarity and humility to keep running, decade after decade, as your body changes and slows down. Actually, it takes humility to do anything over a long period of time and not be discouraged by the ebb and flow of your capacity and level of interest. That's why establishing your intent is so important. So is having a clear commitment and steady discipline. These three elements, along with concentration, mindfulness, and effort, are the necessary ingredients for any long-term practice.

Intent can be defined as a deliberate, clearly formulated resolve or aim. *Commitment* is the wish to achieve that aim. *Discipline* is made up of the actions we take in order to do this. Imagine you're going on a road trip in a foreign country. You've rented a car, bought a map, and plotted your course. Intent is the map. It sets your direction of travel and lets you know when you've wandered off course. Commitment is the wish to get to your destination. Discipline is the fuel you need to travel. Without intent you'll drive around aimlessly, choosing one road and then another. You'll doubt whether the road you've chosen is the right one. You'll switch lanes. You'll speed up, then slow down. Without commitment, you'll get bored or tired of the long journey, wondering when you'll get there. You'll ask yourself if you want to arrive after all. Without discipline, you'll run out of fuel before making it to your destination, then feel guilty or discouraged as car after car passes you by. But if all three elements are present, all you're left with is the practice of driving. One moment after the next, you'll journey on, knowing that travel takes time and persistence.

In the chapters that follow we will explore these elements in greater detail. But for now, I want to encourage you to institute a daily meditation practice if you don't already have one. The instructions I offer here are specifically for zazen. If you already use another form of meditation, consider reviewing this practice anyway. I refer to zazen throughout the book, so becoming familiar with the method will make it easier for you to apply its instructions to running.

Zazen is the heart of the path of self-exploration. Without some form of meditation practice, it is very difficult to see ourselves clearly. So let's start by paring things down to the bare essentials— body, breath, and mind—and on this stable ground build the foundation for a strong running zazen practice.

PRACTICE: STILL SITTING
Establish a daily zazen practice.

To begin, sit on a *zabuton* (a thick cotton mat) and place a *zafu* (a small, round pillow) under you. If you don't have a zabuton and zafu, a blanket and pillow will do. However, if you plan to establish a long-term zazen practice, know that having the appropriate cushions will allow you to sit more comfortably.

When taking your seat, sit cross-legged on the front third of the zafu. This will tilt your pelvis down slightly and allow your knees to come closer to the mat. It will also help to keep your abdomen relaxed so you can breathe freely and naturally.

You can position your legs in different ways. The first and simplest cross-legged pose is the Burmese posture, in which the lower legs are parallel, one in front of the other on the floor in front of you with the tops of the feet resting flat on the mat. Avoid crossing your legs at your ankles and letting your knees dangle in the air—this puts a lot of strain on your back muscles. Sitting higher can help to get your knees closer to the mat, so try turning your cushion on its side and sitting on its top edge, or experiment with different cushions. But if yours knees still don't drop all the way down to the mat, then start with one of the other postures and give your body time to get used to the cross-legged position. Also, stretch whenever you can. I find that doing even ten minutes of yoga or a series of hip-opening exercises every day helps to keep my body limber.

Another cross-legged posture is half lotus, in which one foot (let's say the right) is placed on the left thigh and the left leg is tucked under and behind the right knee. This position is slightly asymmetrical, so you must adjust your sit bones on the cushion in order to avoid leaning to one side. If you use this or the Burmese posture regularly, make a habit of alternating which leg is in front or on top of your other leg to keep your body balanced over time.

The most stable of the postures is full lotus, in which each foot is placed on the opposite thigh, soles of the feet facing up. It's a symmetrical and solid posture, but it's also difficult for most people to do well. In general, I don't recommend starting your zazen practice with it. Most beginners who sit cross-legged use either the Burmese or half-lotus postures if their flexibility allows.

For some people, sitting cross-legged in any of these positions is difficult. An alternative is to kneel on your zabuton in a posture called *seiza*. If you're using a cushion, turn it on its side and straddle it. Make sure you're sitting on the front third and that your abdomen is relaxed. You can also use a specially designed seiza bench, which should be positioned with its tilt facing forward. Kneeling like this helps to take some of the pressure off your ankles, shins, and knees. You can also alternate between the cross-legged and kneeling positions, a practice that is especially helpful during meditation retreats or when sitting for long hours.

If you're not able to sit on the floor, or if you're unsure whether you can do it without moving, consider sitting in a chair. Stillness is paramount in zazen, so make an effort to sit as still as you can, even if you're sitting alone. The reason for this is that every time your body moves, your mind moves, which makes it harder to see what's happening in it. So in zazen, you're letting your body come to rest so your mind can settle.

As you take your seat, be careful not to slump or lean against the chair back, because this is likely to make you drowsy. Ground your body by keeping your feet flat on the floor, and use a zafu or other cushion to support your sit bones. Some people like to use a second back cushion to keep their spine straight, and others sit with no cushion at all. Regardless, make sure that you're not leaning backward. Your posture should support your practice of concentration and wakefulness.

Having chosen your leg position, now allow your back to be straight and your diaphragm to move freely as you breathe. Imagine the top of your head pressing up toward the ceiling, tuck in your chin slightly, and lengthen your spine. Release your shoulders and back muscles, allowing a slight curve in your lower back. The zazen posture is both alert and relaxed. Someone who is sitting well looks immovable, like a mountain. They look as if they've always sat in place, as if they will always sit there, unmoving. It's a posture that is both solid and supple. Firm and soft.

Keep your mouth lightly closed during zazen and breathe naturally through your nose. If you have a cold or your nose is blocked, open your mouth slightly but keep your breath quiet. Softly press your tongue against the upper palate and swallow once to create a seal that will help reduce salivation. This will prevent you from having to swallow constantly.

Your eyes should be open but lowered, with your gaze resting on the ground about two or three feet in front of you. Let your eyelids cover your eyes halfway so you won't have to blink repeatedly. If you've done other kinds of meditation and are used to keeping your eyes closed, you might need to adjust to having your eyes open, but in zazen it's helpful to do this in order to avoid falling asleep.

Rest your hands in your lap. The dominant hand is held palm up under the other hand, also palm up, so that the middle knuckles overlap. Your thumbs should be lightly touching, forming an oval, with your wrists resting on your thighs about two or three fingers' breadth below your navel. This point is called the *hara* in Japanese and the *dantian* in Chinese. It is roughly the center of your body, and it is considered to be the reservoir of your vital energy, or *ki*.

Placing your attention on the hara during zazen will help to quiet your mind and keep you focused.

Now begin counting your breath. With the inhalation, silently count one. Exhale and count two. Inhale, three. Exhale, four. When you get to ten, come back to one. Do this over and over again for as long as you're sitting. In order to build concentration, notice every time your mind begins to wander, and whenever a thought takes you away from your breath, see it, deliberately let it go, and begin counting from one again. It really doesn't matter what the thought is. It could be a profound thought or a mundane thought. It could be the beginning of a song or a reflection on your zazen. Either way, see it clearly, set it aside, and return to counting your breath.

Little by little, your mind will settle. You'll notice you're spending more time actually counting your breath and less time fantasizing or distracting yourself. Your restlessness or boredom or resistance will lessen, and you'll expend less energy to remain present.

Our capacity to concentrate the mind is one of the most powerful traits we have as human beings, yet most of us overlook it. We spend our lives preoccupied with the past or anticipating the future and therefore rarely live in the present. But by deliberately following the three steps outlined above—seeing the thought, letting it go, and returning to the breath—we're training ourselves to keep our attention focused and steady.

In addition to concentration, in zazen you're also developing mindfulness—the ability to see what is in front of you. Gradually you'll learn the difference between a thought that you need to acknowledge and a thought you should put down. Without the constant background buzz of your mind, the thoughts you had wittingly or unwittingly pushed aside or covered up will have space to arise, and it's important not to use zazen to suppress them. If you find that a particular thought recurs no matter how many times you let it go, then shift your practice in order to acknowledge that thought completely. Consciously turn your attention from your breath to that thought and let it fill your mind. Let the thought be present in your awareness without judgment or criticism. You don't have to change it, grab it, or push it away. If you can stay present with it, eventually you'll be able to release it. This sounds simple, but it takes a lifetime of practice to truly let go.

It is said that it takes the mind about twenty minutes to quiet down, so if you can sit longer than that, you will get a taste of the stillness that all of us have access to but so rarely let ourselves touch. If sitting that long seems daunting, then start with five minutes. You can lengthen the time as you become more comfortable with the practice.

Set a timer to track your zazen period so you won't have to constantly check the time. There are a number of apps that offer timed meditation periods, and using one of these can be helpful. Otherwise, a simple timer or your watch's alarm will work just as well.

If you can, sit in the morning as you begin the day and then again before you go to bed at night. Runners often complain that they're too wired to sit still, and so do beginning practitioners. But with time, even the most restless of us can learn to be still. I encourage you to try. The more still you can become, the more likely you are to be awake.

Once zazen becomes an integral part of your life, you'll begin to see how much you normally miss as you rush from one thing to the next, how rarely you are actually present. I remember one morning during breakfast at the monastery I was sitting with a bite of cantaloupe in my mouth, thinking, *I've never really tasted cantaloupe before.* I think this kind of insight is sobering, delightful, and humbling. Sobering because we realize how much we've missed over the years. Delightful because we no longer have to. Humbling because, no matter how much we think we've seen, there is always more to see.

So learn—first through zazen, then through your running—how to move into stillness, since out of this still and fertile ground your ability to live wholeheartedly will grow.

2

Intent

Let's approach this subject of running with a simple question: *Why?* Why do you run? Or, if you haven't yet started, why do you want to? As you answer this question, please take some time to reflect, and be as truthful and deliberate as you can.

Perhaps your answer is that you want to stay in shape as you get older. A reasonable goal. Most of us want to stay in shape as we age. At least, we don't go around thinking, *I hope my body breaks down.* But if you can slow down and look more closely, you might find that "staying in shape" is actually a vague reason to run—not to mention an impractical one. *Which* shape do you want to retain? The one you had when you were eighteen and at your peak form? The shape you had at thirty? At fifty? Or is it actually a shape you've never had but have always wanted?

"Staying in shape" is just a figure of speech, of course. But words create and reflect our views, and these words mirror our strong desire for things to stay the same. We don't like change, and this is especially true when it's happening to our bodies. The problem is, nothing stays in shape for long—not buildings, not mountains, not oceans, and certainly not us.

The building that houses Zen Mountain Monastery was built in the 1920s and '30s as a Benedictine monastery and boys' camp. It's a beautiful structure with bluestone walls and oak beams harvested from the neighboring mountain. There's nothing tenuous about it, nothing fragile. Yet, on closer inspection, you can see that a couple of the beams supporting the floor of what was the chapel and is now a meditation hall have torqued under the weight of thousands of bodies sitting and walking over them. The roof has been replaced in its entirety at least once, and the beautifully laid tiles that used to ripple like waves in the glinting sunlight are now pretty but ordinary. The water cannons that deflect rain off the Zen gardens nestled against the building's front and back façades have rotted and made way for a series of fresh substitutes. And in the meditation hall, a thin crack on the back wall is slowly, quietly, and inexorably splitting the building apart. Every time I look at the gap I wonder what the monastery will look like a century or two from now.

For each of us, the process of decay happens much quicker. Our skin sags, our cheeks droop, hard spots go soft, bones get dry and brittle. No matter how hard we labor against aging, how much we resist it, we can't avoid the fact that it is not a manufacturing defect. Our bodies are supposed to wear out and eventually fall apart. They will do so literally, as the aggregates that constitute what we call body and mind, life and consciousness actually come apart in the dying process. So regardless of how much time, effort, or money we devote to staying in shape, not a single one of us will succeed in doing so for long.

But maybe you're not yet concerned about getting old. Maybe your reason for running is that you want to be healthy. Another sensible goal. Now ask yourself: what does being healthy mean to you, and what do you need to maintain that state? Is running two or three times a week for half an hour enough, or do you feel you need to run at least six miles a day, five times a week? What happens when you miss a day or two, or more? Do you feel anxious that your health is slipping?

The wellness industry is a trillion-dollar market in the United States, and it is fueled by our obsession with health and our fear of aging and death. But what *is* health? Is it just the absence of sickness? Or is it the same as weight loss and fitness? How does being healthy relate to living a balanced life?

Besides health and fitness, there are many reasons to run, conscious or not. The practice of defining your intent makes these reasons apparent. So as you continue reading, consider whether any of these motivations reflect your own. Or perhaps there is something else driving you. Either way, engage in the process of inquiry—this is the most important aspect of working with your intent.

Running as Escape

Some people run to get away from something: a tortured past, an addiction, a broken heart. Running can be good medicine, but in itself it is rarely a cure. If you run to stay away from drugs, for example, that is certainly a worthwhile intent. Running can be a powerful balm for the pain that leads any of us to seek solace in drugs, alcohol, food, or television—just a few of all possible addictions. When my mother died, it was running that helped me to hold and move through my body the grief that at times threatened to overwhelm me. But by itself, running didn't address the source of my pain. Unless we find a way to face and work with our feelings, running can become just another kind of drug.

During my late teens I went through a period of what I can only describe as obsessive running. In retrospect I can see I was finding it hard to be with myself (who doesn't at that age?) and running kept me from feeling what I couldn't bear to feel. I ran and ran, and although I could sense it had become a kind of addiction, I was unable to stop. I felt good when I ran. Strong and powerful. Focused and in control. And I could justify my excessive running by telling myself it isn't harmful like drugs. So I kept going.

But like any other addiction, eventually my obsession caught up with me. Gradually I began to feel tired, then resistant. I wanted to do other things besides running, but I never had the time or energy. I thought of pulling back. I thought of quitting, but I was too proud. Besides, what was a little resistance? I'd felt it before and knew how to get through it: push harder, and don't think too much. I ran even harder and longer.

One day I was in a car going somewhere. I don't remember whom I was with or where I was headed, but I have a vivid image of what I saw through the window: It was a beautiful fall day, cool and sunny. Young couples were leisurely walking arm in arm, shaggy-haired students with backpacks slung over their shoulders ambled down the sidewalk, passing by nannies pushing their strollers. The maples, oaks, and birches were bursting with blood red, ocher, and gold—an orgy of Byzantine color. Normally I would have been delighted in the display, but that afternoon I couldn't care less. I sat slumped in the backseat, glaring at the people strolling by, thinking, *They don't have to run.* And I hated them. I hated these strangers who could do as they pleased, who clearly felt no need to run and seemed perfectly content about it. *How dare they?*

My resentment was visceral. It was complete.

A part of me could see the ridiculousness of my situation. No one had forced me to run. I wasn't training for a race. I wasn't even part of a running club or group that depended on my commitment. I was the only one who'd patiently built my cell, laying brick on top of brick. I'd carefully installed the padlock, and I'd swallowed the key. Now I was hollering at the passersby for turning me into a prisoner. Still, I couldn't shift. I was like a machine caught in a loop. Two days later, I was running again.

I kept this up until I developed tendonitis so severe I could barely walk. And for the two months that it took to heal, instead of reflecting on why I'd been so manic, I spent my free time swimming and riding a stationary bicycle, terrified that if I let too much time pass without exercising, my body would break down.

It wasn't until I started doing zazen a couple of years later that I was able to see this pattern. Eventually I was able to recognize the difference between running for pleasure and running as escape, and over time I developed the skills to cope with my feelings more effectively. In addition, I came to see that I was both afraid of my body and afraid of losing control. It took many years of practice, but in the end I was able to get to the point where I could run just for the sake of running—for the simple joy of moving my body. Still, on occasion I do wonder if, without a spiritual practice, I would still be running from myself.

Running for Dear Life

Some people run toward something, like a second chance. When a friend of mine was only seventeen, she was hit by a car while riding her bike. Soon after, her doctors told her she might never be able to walk again. Undaunted, she decided that running would become her therapy. She joined a track team and gradually worked her way up from limping to walking to jogging. After a few years, she was one of the team's long-distance runners. Running literally saved her, and although thirty years later she no longer runs, she still feels immense gratitude for the gift that it gave her.

Some people run to challenge themselves. Some run to strengthen their sense of self-worth, or out of longing to be wanted and loved. A few do it simply because they love it and nothing else.

But it's also possible that some of us run out of the primal fear of death that we are all prey to. The writer and runner Haruki Murakami once said that runners run to live their lives to the fullest, not out of a desire to live longer. I think this is true to some extent. Yet I also think that we can use running—or any other sport—to repress that most inconvenient fact of a human life: that it ends. We all know we're going to die, but we don't really want to know it. Our desire to *be* is the most powerful force there is, only equivalent to our fear of dying. Knowing this is true won't save us from death, but it might make coping with it a little easier.

Tibetan Buddhist teachers say it like it is: all of us are going to die, and the purpose of spiritual practice is to prepare us for the process. So although I'm not implying that all runners run out of existential fear, I do think we cannot discount the anxiety that many of us operate from—an anxiety that takes many forms and often permeates our actions, especially when it remains unacknowledged.

Ask yourself, if you knew you could live forever, would you still run? Or would you run as much as you do now? If the answer to both questions is yes, then not only do you run because you truly love it, you're also free of the multilayered fear that compels many of us to exercise. Fear of illness, of aging, of death. Fear of losing our looks, our vitality, our strength. Fear of our vulnerability, our humanity, our ordinariness. Fear of fading from the memory of others.

Use your running practice, then, to see yourself more clearly—to understand what drives you. But don't force the process. Deep inquiry requires silence, stillness, and patience. The paradox of still running is that you have to learn to slow down even while moving quickly.

PRACTICE: WHY DO YOU RUN?

*Set aside 10 to 15 minutes to clarify
your intent for running.*

Before you go out for your next run, spend a few minutes doing this practice, and return to it periodically, especially if you find yourself in a running slump. We find time, energy, and resources to do the things we love. Is running one of them? If so, then what's stopping you? Or are you finding you don't actually want to run anymore? That's fine. You can drop it without guilt and turn your attention and energy to the things you really want to do. Running zazen is about uncovering what is true, even if that means letting go of running itself.

You can do this practice alone, or if you have a running partner, go through it together. Sometimes speaking your intent aloud can help to clarify feelings you didn't even know you had. Another option is to keep a journal of these practices. If you're used to maintaining a running journal, this won't be a stretch for you. But rather than focusing on the externals of your running regimen—the miles you've logged, the food you've eaten, the shoes you've bought—you'll use writing to observe and record your experience of the act of running. Be as detailed and specific as you can. Note your reactions to each of the practices, even—or especially—if they're negative. Is there a particular practice that doesn't work for you? Are you feeling resistant? Do you struggle to follow the instructions? Why?

No one needs to read this journal, so the more honest you can be as you're writing, the more useful it will be to you. Remember that you're engaging zazen and still running in order to know yourself more clearly, and there are few things that teach us more than those that make us bristle.

When you're ready to begin, start with the fundamental question: why? Out of all the many activities you could do in your free time, why choose running? What do you want to get out of it, if anything? If you've been running for a while, is your intent the same as when you first started? Are you doing what you said you were going to do? If not, why not? Again, be less concerned about facts—you haven't run as often or as long as you said you would, for example—and more about the reasons behind your choices. Use these questions to clarify your running practice, but remember that you can also use this process to explore the why and how of anything that you do.

The thirteenth-century Japanese Zen master Dogen said: "When one gains one dharma, one penetrates one dharma; when one encounters one action, one practices one action." In Buddhism, *dharma* means natural order, truth, or phenomenon. It also refers to the body of the Buddha's teachings. So think of running as the one dharma in front of you. If you can penetrate and understand running, there's no reason you cannot do the same when a different dharma presents itself to you. So whether you're running or working, know why you do what you do, and allow yourself to meet each activity wholeheartedly.

3

Commitment

At the end of the fall training period, a young monk stands outside his teacher's room, collecting himself. He has spent twenty years studying with the great Chinese Zen master Moshan Liaoran, known far and wide for her clarity and fierceness. Now, having finished his training, he's ready to set off on his own. But he's nervous. He knows he might not see Moshan again, and he's worried about what her last teaching to him might be. She's never been one to mince words.

The monk takes a deep breath. Then he removes his sandals, places them neatly on the floor next to the door, and shakes out the umbrella he is carrying. He sets that down also and carefully arranges his robes before knocking on the door.

"Come in," Moshan says.

The monk opens the door, does three bows at the threshold of the room, and stands respectfully in front of his teacher, his hands palm to palm in *gassho*, a gesture of gratitude and reverence.

Moshan regards her student quietly.

"Is it raining outside?" she asks after a moment.

"Oh, yes. It's raining quite hard," the monk says with relief. Maybe she'll go easy on him after all.

Moshan nods. "Did you bring an umbrella?"

"Yes. I left it on the stoop."

"I see," says Moshan. She pauses again. "And did you leave it to the right or to the left of your sandals?"

The monk stands dumbfounded while Moshan waits patiently. Outside, the rain is falling in sheets, soaking the rice fields. *To the right or to the left?* The monk racks his brain but cannot come up with an answer. Another moment passes. He opens his mouth, closes it, then turns and goes back into the meditation hall.

Ten years later, he was still studying with Master Moshan.

I've told this story to many audiences of prospective Zen students, and every once in a while one of them will come up to me to express their alarm. "If this is the kind of commitment required to study Zen, I don't think I have it," they'll say. Perhaps. But as with any other aspect of practice, there's a whole range within which commitment operates, and we shortchange ourselves when we anticipate limits that may not actually be there.

There are various way to think about commitment: as a vow, resolution, promise, duty, or tie. As it relates to practice and intent, commitment is a firm decision to do what we say we want to do. It is the glue that binds together intent and discipline.

Many of us struggle with commitment. Yet I believe that our difficulty stems less from our inability to follow through on our choices than from our lack of clarity about what we want. When our intent is muddled, our commitment easily wavers. But when our intent is strong and clear, we become unshakable.

Diana Nyad was sixty-four when she stepped ashore in Key West after swimming for fifty-three hours continuously. It was her fifth attempt to do the Cuba–Florida crossing, a goal fueled by what she called the "thrill of commitment." And while few of us have the desire to follow either the monk's or Nyad's example, all of us can benefit from exploring our commitments, large and small.

Commitment, like practice, requires clarity, concentration, consistency, and courage. This is true whether we're chasing a lifelong dream or just trying to establish a running practice. Each of us meets our commitments where we are, in accordance with our capacity and aspiration. When that commitment matches our intent, our practice can proceed more smoothly. And if our commitment needs to change to match a new intent, knowing this makes it possible to adjust accordingly.

Let me give you an example. If you want to boil a pot of water, first you have to identify the elements you absolutely need: a heat source, water, and a pot. These are the essential ingredients required to see through your intent. Other elements—a big kitchen, background music, a nice view—are pleasant but extraneous. Also extraneous are your opinions, beliefs, and feelings about water. Water will boil when it reaches the right temperature, whether you like this fact, feel conflicted about it, or disagree with it on principle. And while this doesn't mean your feelings are unimportant, it is helpful to know if and how they might affect your commitment.

While at the monastery, I learned this simple but powerful lesson. Every morning and every evening the residents were expected to be in the zendo for the scheduled hour and a half of zazen, regardless of whether we felt up for it or not. Since our days were long and often included physical labor, it wasn't unusual for one or more of us to feel too tired to sit quietly without dozing off. This was certainly the case for me. Dawn is my favorite time of day, so I had no qualms about getting up early to sit. But evening zazen was torture. By eight o'clock at night I was so exhausted that I could barely stay upright on my cushion, let alone concentrate. Yet my commitment was to be present for both blocks of zazen. I could fight this fact, or I could accept it. After a while, it dawned on me that my dislike of night sitting did not have to impede the zazen itself. I told myself that, instead of trying to focus as strongly as I did in the morning, I would just sit as still and quietly as I could. And just like that, evening zazen stopped being such a struggle. I still preferred to sit early in the day, but since I was no longer fighting myself, I didn't feel so depleted.

Once you've identified the main ingredients to fulfill your intent, you'll need to train yourself to focus on what you're doing and then sustain that focus over time. If you turn off the flame as the water is starting to get hot, or if every few minutes you move the pot to a different burner, you'll never have boiling water. This is the practice of applying concentration and consistency, both of which undoubtedly take effort. But as we'll see, the right kind of effort feeds on itself. The more we concentrate, the more we're able to concentrate. The inverse is also true. We often expend large amounts of energy on tangents either loosely related or completely unconnected to our original intent, and then we become discouraged when we get distracted or lose our momentum.

It's also important to know that, just as we cannot control the way water molecules respond to heat or the speed at which they reach their boiling point, we cannot force circumstances to conform to our commitment. But we can study that commitment carefully in order to discern whether the elements of clarity, concentration, consistency, and—in the case of more significant endeavors—courage, are in place to help us see it through.

Clarity: Seeing Things as They Are

Earlier I said that the study of reality is the study of things as they are. In Buddhism this is called realizing enlightenment, or "suchness." But the reason it is so challenging to perceive clearly is that we normally see through what Buddhist philosophy calls the realms of images and representations. We see our ideas, dreams, and symbols of reality—not reality itself. Even Western philosophy makes a distinction between direct and indirect perception. Immanuel Kant said that we can never really be sure that things are as we perceive them to be, because what we see is always filtered through the mind. A "thing-in-itself," or *noumenon*, can never be known, he said. We can only perceive the *phenomenon*, the "thing-as-it-appears." But the fact is, we *can* see things clearly and directly. This is what the Buddha realized 2,500 years ago. It is what generations of Buddhist teachers have reiterated since. In order to see in this way, we must clear the filters that often distort our perception of reality—our beliefs, ideas, judgments, and preconceived notions.

In a sutra called the *Tittha Sutta*, the Buddha teaches his monks about the importance of not attaching to views, and as an example, he tells them the story of the blind men and the elephant. "Once there was a king in the city of Shravasti," the Buddha said. "The king asked that an elephant be presented to a group of blind men so they could become acquainted with this great animal. When the elephant was brought before them, each of the men touched a part of its enormous body: one felt the head, another the ear, another the tusk, the trunk, the body, the foot, the hindquarters, the tail, and the tail tuft. Afterward, the king asked his subjects what an elephant was like. The first man said, 'An elephant is like a water jar.' The second said it was like a winnowing basket. The third, a plowshare. A plow pole. A storeroom. A post. A mortar. A pestle. A broom."

The Buddha then said to his monks, "Just so, wanderers travel around, saying, 'The truth is like this,' 'The truth is like that,' but they are all blind."

Our own seeing is often like this. We see only partially, or we determine what we're seeing based on our feelings, opinions, or memories. And while none of us can be completely free of these filters, knowing that they are in place can help us to see through them. Zazen, with its emphasis on stillness and concentration, is a powerful tool for facilitating this type of direct seeing. It allows us to go beyond the "thing-as-it-appears" to see the "thing-in-itself." This is what in Buddhism we call clarity or insight.

Concentration: Ignoring the Nonessentials

A stable and focused mind is the cornerstone of any meditative practice. In order to see, we must first be able to concentrate. Soma Thera, the late Sinhalese Buddhist monk and scholar, spoke of concentration in the following way: "One plants one's consciousness deep in an object like a firm post well sunk in the ground, and withstands the tempestuous clamor of the extraneous by a sublime ignoring of non-essentials."

In order to gain insight, we must withstand the onslaught of all the many sights and sounds and thoughts that get in the way of our concentration. This "ignoring of non-essentials" is sublime, however, because it's in the service of our clarity. Likewise, when establishing a zazen or running practice, we ignore the non-essentials so we can focus on the indispensable. We keep things simple and limited—at least for the duration of the task we're trying to accomplish.

The dancer and choreographer Twyla Tharp has said that, while she's working on a project, she cuts out all distractions. She doesn't look at anything with numbers (clocks, bills, or scales), watch movies, listen to music not pertaining to her work, or do any type of multitasking. This kind of disciplined focus is Tharp's temporary renunciation of the non-essentials to free up her time and mental space for the demanding task of creation.

Anyone who's ever attempted to master an art form knows that commitment and discipline are integral to the process. I don't know if this story is apocryphal, but I once read that the writer Don DeLillo used to strap himself to his desk chair with the belt of his bathrobe to keep himself working during a writing session. In zazen, we do the equivalent by not moving. No matter how tired, distracted, or restless we feel, we commit to staying put until the period is over, renouncing the impulse to move away from our discomfort. Because when we shift too quickly in order to avoid our unease, we miss the opportunity to see that, just beyond the boundary of what we can see, past the edge of what we know, lies a world of possibility.

There's a story of a four-year-old girl who was engrossed in a school art project. Her teacher watched her with interest as one hour, then two went by and the girl did not budge from her seat.

Finally the teacher approached the child and said, "Lily, I see you've been very busy drawing something. Can you tell me what it is?"

"I'm drawing God," Lily said, without looking up from her work.

"But no one has ever seen God," the teacher said, amused.

Lily looked up and caught her teacher's eye. "They will in a minute."

Focus and consistency make it possible for us to push against the edges of what we think we know. They allow us to take the risks necessary to fulfill the wish we have expressed by our commitment and discover what is yet unrevealed. But commitment is not the same as certainty. The risk we're taking would not be a risk if we could know the outcome beforehand. So commitment requires that we believe deeply in our intent, even though ultimately we don't know whether we will succeed or not. Nyad could have failed a fifth time. DeLillo might have lacked the talent for writing, Tharp for dancing. Yet I suspect that, even at those times when they most doubted themselves, their courage still exceeded their hesitation.

Courage: Living Wholeheartedly

Any long-term commitment will at some point demand that we stretch beyond our current limits. That is why a certain amount of daring, a willingness to challenge ourselves to go beyond our realm of comfort, is necessary.

A fellow runner once told me she wanted to run a race in every town in her state.

"Why?" I asked her.

She thought for a while before answering. "To know that I've done it. To challenge myself."

Part of me wanted to press her further and ask why it was important for her to do this. Yet I also understood the impulse. It's the same drive that makes a casual runner begin training for a marathon or that compels an ultramarathoner to run longer distances. It's the thrill—as Nyad said—that pushes us to challenge ourselves beyond our own ideas of who we are and what we think we're capable of.

I believe we do want to live our lives wholeheartedly, as Murakami said. But we don't have to go out of our way to force this sense of aliveness. Practice shows us that we can find fulfillment even within the most ordinary activities, that there is inherent wonder and majesty in the humblest of things.

One of my favorite Zen koans describes a dialogue between two monks, Dongshan and Shenshan, who would eventually become great dharma teachers during the heyday of Zen in Tang Dynasty China.

Early one morning, Shenshan was patching his robes. Dongshan passed by, and seeing his dharma brother bent over his sewing table, he asked, "What are you doing?"

Shenshan said, "I'm sewing."

Dongshan probed a little further. "What is sewing?"

"Each stitch follows the other," said Shenshan. A standard Zen answer. We do one stitch, then another, then another. As Master Dogen said, we meet each dharma as it presents itself to us. But Dongshan was not satisfied.

"If you say so," he shrugged and started to walk away.

"What would you say?" Shenshan asked.

Dongshan turned to face Shenshan. "Each stitch is like the earth exploding."

Each stitch, each step, each action, is like the whole world exploding. Do you know what Dongshan means? His statement is a living expression of wholeheartedness—another word for deep commitment. Dongshan is not concerned with the task of sewing. He's not thinking about the robe or about this or that stitch, about before or after. He fully understands that each stitch is so complete, so all-encompassing, that it includes the robe, him, Shenshan, and the entire world. So when a single stitch is sewn, the earth dies with it. With the next stitch, the earth is born again, and again it explodes. Moment by moment, the whole of reality is created.

To sew with wakefulness, to listen to your child as if each word were her first and last, to run as if each step you take is the only one—this is what it means to live with courage and wholeheartedness. Yet there is more to courage than bravery. In the context of the spiritual path, courage rests on one of the central tenets of Buddhism: our original perfection.

Perfect as We Are

"Success is stumbling from failure to failure with no loss of enthusiasm," Winston Churchill once said. Willingness to fail is an integral aspect of commitment, and although intellectually most of us know that we can't expect to succeed without failing on occasion, we are usually so failure-averse that we're willing to remain in lukewarm, unsatisfying, or even harmful situations in order to avoid the risk of failing in new territory.

"But that's normal," a friend said to me when I told him I was writing this chapter. "I only like to do things in which I excel. I don't like to fail. Nobody does."

True, but how do we learn and grow without the time, energy, and repeated failures that inevitably result when we stretch ourselves beyond our capacity? And what is failure, anyway?

A couple of years ago I gave a talk on Zen Buddhism to a group of about a hundred people in New York City. I'd spoken before this audience in the past and had felt that their response to my talks was generally positive. But this time a woman in the back began dozing almost immediately after I began speaking, and halfway through my talk she actually fell off her chair, creating a small commotion. Afterward she came up to me and sheepishly said she was worn out that morning, but she assured me that she had loved my presentation. I knew better. I can usually sense when I have an audience's attention, and this time I was certain I had lost them early on. So I suspected she was simply embodying what the rest of the audience must have been feeling. I thanked her and scurried off with my tail between my legs, then spent the next few hours feeling mortified. Shame and self-doubt flooded my mind, thoughts I was certain I'd left behind long ago, given my years of practice. *Who do you think you are, believing you can do this? Clearly you're not cut out for public speaking—and now everyone knows it. What a terrible talk!* I tried to reason with these minor demons, arguing that I hadn't hurt or insulted anyone. In the scheme of things, a bad talk was unimportant, I told myself. Most likely, those present that morning had already forgotten what I'd said. Still, it was hard to let go of my shame. It felt significant and thoroughly discomfiting. Then it occurred to me that there might be another way for me to look at this "failure."

The Buddha, perhaps surprisingly, spoke of shame as a skillful emotion. Paired with fear of wrongdoing, he called it a "bright principle" that protects the world from our potentially harmful actions. In Pali, *hiri* is the internal shame we feel at losing our sense of honor or self-respect. *Ottappa* is the external fear of the consequences of our unskillful or hurtful actions, including the effect they might have on others. In a graphic analogy, Buddhaghosa, a fifth-century Theravada Buddhist monk, likened hiri and ottappa to the reactions we'd have were we to grab either end of an iron rod smeared with excrement on one side and heated to a red-hot glow on the other. Shame, he said, is the disgust we'd feel at grasping the side covered with excrement. Fear of wrongdoing is the pain and distress we'd experience from holding the hot side of the rod. Both feelings are extremely uncomfortable and depending on the offense, perhaps intolerable. But it is that very discomfort that alerts us to the fact that there is something we need to attend to, something we need to rectify.

As I reflected on my own feeling of shame, I realized that I was taking the woman's boredom as a reflection of my worth as a speaker—and worse, of my worth as a person. But this is a Western misunderstanding of the feeling of shame, which translates into the thoughts *There is something wrong with me* and *I'm unworthy.* Yet, shame as a bright principle is not supposed to cause us suffering; it's meant to alleviate it. The Buddha said shame is skillful because it throws our actions into question. It makes us wonder whether we could have responded to the circumstances with greater harmony, but it never raises any doubts about our worth.

Buddhism states that every being, from the moment of inception, is originally perfect and complete, lacking nothing. Inherently we are in full possession of every quality and every virtue we require to realize who we are and to live our lives accordingly. However, perfection is not infallibility. It is not perfectionism, and it is not flawlessness.

The word *perfection* comes from the Latin noun *perfectio* and the adjective *perfectus*, both of which are derived from the verb *perficere*, "to complete." So perfection is tantamount to wholeness, completeness, and—to use the Buddhist concept—suchness. Something is perfect simply because it *is*. It is perfect *just* as it is, mistakes and flaws included.

In the *Metaphysics*, Aristotle said that a thing can be called perfect or complete when nothing can be found outside of it. In other words, there isn't anything this completeness does not admit. Many centuries later, Master Dogen used similar language to describe this original perfection: "No creature ever falls short of its own completeness. Wherever it stands, it never fails to cover the ground." But we don't know, and therefore don't act from, this truth. That is why we need practice and realization.

In my own innocuous example, the woman's boredom was not a reflection of anything other than my need to improve my ability as a speaker. I wasn't bad or flawed or unworthy. I simply still had work to do. There were certain skills I still needed to learn, which is true of all aspects of my life—professional, psychological, and spiritual. My anger, my selfishness, my impatience, my blindness are all signs of both my humanity and my potential for further growth.

Despite original perfection, none of us come out of the womb as fully realized buddhas. In the words of Shunryu Suzuki Roshi, one of the pioneer Japanese teachers who brought Zen to the West, "Each of you is perfect the way you are . . . and you can use a little improvement." Insight helps us to see our original perfection. Practice is the process of developing it so it can function in our lives.

Thankfully, the spiritual path does not conform to our usual measures of success and failure. Neither does life. Every time we "fail" we are presented with yet another opportunity to see ourselves more clearly, and to integrate that insight more fully. Practice doesn't end. But this is the good news of Buddhism, because in practice and commitment, there is no arrival apart from the present moment.

PRACTICE: RUNNING WITH CONSISTENCY

Commit to a consistent running practice
for a minimum of a month.

If you have difficulty with commitment, this practice is especially important for you. Take some time to determine how much and how often you want to run, and then make an agreement with yourself to follow your intent for a month. Write it down in your own words, and don't be afraid to express it as an actual commitment. For example: "I commit to run three miles a day, three days a week, for a month." Below it, write down your intent for doing this, and as always, be as specific as you can. Sign the agreement, and post it on your refrigerator door or somewhere where you'll be able to see it. Refer to it when you forget or feel ambivalent about the promise you made to yourself.

Whatever your commitment, let it stretch you just beyond your current limits, but be reasonable. It's better to start slowly and build on your commitment than to set yourself up for disappointment. If you live with others, talk to them and explain what you want to do (this is also helpful when establishing a daily sitting practice). If necessary, negotiate. Then use your journal to keep track of your commitment. If, as the month progresses, you miss any running days, don't be shy about noting them so you will have an accurate assessment of your progress over the course of the month. Don't worry about failure, and don't berate yourself for not fulfilling your promise. More than anything, this is a practice of discernment. You are learning, in real time, how much running is both sustainable and desirable for you. So do not see this practice as an obligation. Instead, consider it as an opportunity to learn what it is that you actually want and are able to do. If you find yourself slipping, return to your commitment and let it guide you through the end of the month. Once the thirty days are over, assess what happened.

Were you able to keep your commitment as you set it down? If not, why not? Can you identify the obstacles? Could you have done anything differently to avoid or work through them? On the other hand, could you have run more? If the answer is yes, consider renewing your commitment, increasing the frequency or distance of your runs. Again, be conservative. But remember that your limits are never fixed or static. *You* are never fixed or static, so don't be afraid of challenging yourself. That's the only way you'll find out the kind of power you inherently possess.

4

Discipline

Let's face it—discipline is not a popular concept. For many of us, the term evokes images of pursed lips and wagging fingers, compulsory lessons, and enforced quiet time or, later in life, mandatory labor and punishment. When I looked up the word in half a dozen dictionaries, their definitions only solidified these associations. I read that discipline is "the practice of training people to obey rules or a code of behavior, using punishment to correct disobedience," "penitential chastisement," and "physical punishment, teaching, suffering, martyrdom." Less punitively but not any more lightly, discipline is also defined as "training that corrects, molds, or perfects the mental faculties or moral character" and "a rule or system of rules governing conduct or activity."

The original meaning of the Latin *disciplina* was "instruction given, teaching, learning, knowledge," but sometime in the Middle Ages the term took on the connotation of punishment and even "mortification by scourging." (Indeed, the sentence given as an example under the definition for *connotation* in the *New Oxford American Dictionary* reads, "The word *discipline* has unhappy connotations of punishment and repression.")

Unequivocally, our use of the term has firmly established discipline as the polar opposite of enjoyment. Discipline is the bitter medicine we must gulp down because it's "good for us"—because it will either help us accomplish a goal or give the sense of strength we so crave and wish to preserve. From this perspective, being disciplined means forcing ourselves to do what we have to do. But this kind of discipline is externally compelled and thus precarious.

There is another way to think about discipline, however, and that is as self-empowerment. As *wanting* to do what we have to do. In this case, being disciplined means exercising full power within our lives. It means choosing our actions according to a deep desire and a carefully thought-out motivation, instead of a sense of obligation or a fear of consequences. When we act in a disciplined way, we are expressing our wish for our actions to be in harmony with both our intent and our commitment. We are saying we want to pair what we say with what we do.

There is a story about Mahatma Gandhi that illustrates this view of discipline.

A young Indian mother was concerned about the amount of sugar her son ate. The boy happily binged on pastries, soft drinks, ice cream, and candy, and nothing his mother tried succeeded in curbing his sweet tooth. But then she had an idea. She set off with her son on the long trip from the coast to Gujarat to see Mahatma Gandhi.

"Gandhiji, my son eats too much sugar," she said when she had been admitted to see the great master. "I'm very worried about his health, but he won't listen to me. Yet he respects you greatly, and I think if you spoke to him, he might stop. Please, will you tell him it is bad for him to eat this way?"

Gandhi pondered her request, then asked that the two of them return a week later. Crestfallen, the woman mumbled her agreement and went outside to meet her son. Back they went the way they had come, only to return a week later. This time Gandhi asked that they both see him together.

They entered the room shyly, the boy hiding behind his mother's sari. Gandhi gestured to the boy to get close. Reluctantly he came forward, his gaze on the ground. When he was only a few feet from the Mahatma, Gandhi smiled brightly at him.

"My son," he said, "you should not eat sugar anymore. It's bad for your health."

The boy nodded and ran back to his mother, who struggled for a moment to hide her annoyance.

"But Gandhiji," she finally said, "why didn't you just say this to him last week?"

Gandhi adjusted his glasses and smiled again, this time with a trace of bashfulness. "Because last week I was eating too much sugar myself."

When Your Wish Becomes an Imperative

Given a choice, most of us will do what we want and avoid what we don't. Even when pressed to do things we'd rather avoid, we're infinitely creative at finding ways to subvert the process. We get sick, we procrastinate, we silently or overtly rebel. The more choices we have, the less likely we are to respond to coercion—especially coming from ourselves. The ego loves insurrection and is happy to fight even itself to get attention.

Who hasn't had the experience of firmly stating an intent only to turn around and do the very opposite? Growing up, I had a neighbor who was perpetually following the latest diet fad. But the more extreme the regimen, the more blatantly she broke it. "I'm not eating dairy," she'd say, and a day later I'd find her on her stoop having a pint of frozen yogurt. "This?" she'd innocently ask when I referenced her ban on dairy. "This doesn't count. It's not real ice cream."

We call this kind of rebellion self-sabotage, but I think it's actually self-preservation, for conflict is the ideal way for the self to remain center stage. As long as we are mired in the tension between "I should" and "I want," our minds stay occupied with arguments, excuses, and justifications. We become our own judge and jury. We act as defendant, plaintiff, prosecutor, and defense. Busy with our own trial, we're busy with *ourselves*—which is exactly what the self wants. It doesn't want to be forgotten, and it will do anything to keep itself alive.

"I want to run a marathon," someone said to me after attending one of my running retreats. "The problem is, I lack the discipline. I just don't seem to be able to get over my resistance at having to wake up early in order to train."

"Well, *why* do you want to run a marathon?" I asked him.

"I want to push myself," the man said. "I want to do something that I haven't done before."

I pointed out to him that this intent was too vague to establish a viable discipline. "When your alarm goes off to tell you it's time for your early morning run, and it's thirty degrees and pitch black outside," I said, "'I want to push myself' may not be a strong enough reason to get you out of bed." I explained that, unless he grounded his actions on a clearer intent, he'd easily lose interest. The key, I added, is to see discipline as a matter of choice and self-power. If he could get to a place where he was choosing to get out of bed in order to fulfill his intent for running, then his discipline would follow. I said, "Choose to do what you have to do."

Based on this perspective, let me offer my own working definition of discipline: the practice of training yourself to identify what is most important to you, and the careful and persistent work of choosing actions that support that aim.

John Muir, founder of the Sierra Club, grew up on a farm with a father who thought his children should always be occupied in one of two ways: working or reading the Bible. But Muir had a curious, restless mind. He loved reading all kinds of books and inventing things—activities his father rejected as wastes of time. But one night Muir woke up accidentally around one in the morning and realized that he had five solid hours before he had to begin his daily chores. So he decided he'd wake up at that time every night to read and tinker to his heart's content. Then, to help himself, he invented a special alarm clock: at the appointed time, the mechanism—

which was rigged to Muir's bed—would flip the mattress vertically, setting him on his feet. It also lit a candle and opened his book to the page where he'd stopped reading the night before.

Not all of us have Muir's resoluteness or ingenuity. But like our commitment, we can establish our discipline in the form and to the degree that is accessible to us. Basing that commitment and discipline on our intent, we chart—if not an easy course, necessarily—a clearer path.

Returning to the man's wish to run a marathon, let's examine how he could investigate the relationship between his intent, commitment, and discipline.

First he would state his intent as clearly as possible. "I want to run a marathon because it's important to me to challenge myself. I want to move beyond my comfort zone in order to build self-confidence," might be one formulation. Or "I want to raise money for leukemia research," or "I need a way to be more connected to my body and the natural world. I spend too many hours sitting in an office."

Second, he would work to identify the most skillful means to fulfill that intent. In Buddhism, *skillful means*, or *upaya*, refers to an enlightened teacher's ability to teach the dharma. More generally, it is the means by which we bring our intent to fruition through the process of practice. So for our fellow runner, the skillful means to achieve his intent to train for a marathon might include joining a running club, buying books about marathon running, or hiring a coach.

Third, he would need to discern whether these means are actually skillful—not just for him but also for those around him and the circumstances in which he finds himself.

During a retreat I offered on the topic of discipline in Buddhist practice, one of the participants told me he had a friend who had never missed a day at the gym over the past ten years. "He's in great shape, as you can imagine," the man said. "But he's not an easy person to be around." I nodded, knowing from experience what he meant. I said that, in all likelihood, flexibility and compromise were not his friend's strongest qualities. Then I pointed out that this is the view of discipline most of us hold: we do what we have to do, no matter the cost.

But as we engage in spiritual practice, how do we balance our own desires with those of others? Any form of discipline requires time, focus, and energy. How do we widen that focus to take in the people we affect with our actions? This is a challenging and delicate balance.

Fourth, our runner would examine whether he was able to accomplish his intent. Having started a training regimen, did he find himself skipping days or cheating on his workouts? Did he follow the program religiously, even though he didn't really enjoy it? Or was he able to remain flexible yet committed? When he actually ran the race, did he feel a sense of accomplishment, or only relief at having finished?

We make choices based on our understanding of our actions and their results. So as you consider the discipline required to maintain a running practice, turn to those actions that remind you of your intent and that support your commitment. *Choose* to do what you *have* to do. Or, conversely, strengthen your intent such that you'll *have* to do what you *want* to do. Allow your wish to become an imperative.

Remember, you can think of discipline as restraint, or you can see it as choice. And the clearer your understanding about the relationship between thought and action, the easier it will be to make that choice.

Our Actions Are Our Belongings

According to an early Buddhist philosophical school called the Yogachara, consciousness is divided into eight different types. The first six are the six sense consciousnesses: eye, ear, nose, tongue, body, and mind. Usually we think of only the first five as the senses through which we perceive the world, but in Buddhism mind is also a sense, and its object is thought. The mind's job is to take information from the other five senses and filter it through *manas*, the seventh consciousness, which roughly corresponds to the Western concept of ego or self. Manas is the "me" that perceives, senses, thinks, and cognizes. It is also our survival instinct, our sense of self-preservation. Underlying all of these is the eighth consciousness, the *alaya-vijñana*, or storehouse consciousness. In this foundational consciousness are stored all the "seeds" of every action we have ever experienced or perceived, and these seeds have the potential to "bloom" into events in our experience.

Commenting on this teaching, Thich Nhat Hanh says that mind consciousness is like a gardener, and the storehouse consciousness is its garden. Depending on the seeds we choose to water, certain actions will bloom and become results, while others will lie fallow. Every time our runner friend chooses to get up early to train, he increases the probability of doing it again the following morning. His actions are watering the seeds of a daily running practice. On the other hand, the more days he skips—the longer he lets the soil dry out between runs—the harder he'll have to work to bring those seeds back to life.

Every action is consistent with its result. As gardeners we would never plant a lemon seed in the hope that it would grow into an apple tree. Yet in our lives, we don't hesitate to feed our negative thoughts but are surprised that we feel so unhappy.

My teacher used to invoke the following thought experiment. Imagine two individuals whose lives are fundamentally satisfying. They both have families, jobs, food, safety, and some degree of leisure. One of them is asked to spend the first hour of her day bringing to mind everything she is dissatisfied with in her life, while the other must fill the same amount of time with expressions of gratitude. Day after day they do this, repeating the same ritual for a whole year. "When the time is up, whom do you think you will want to spend time with?" my teacher would ask.

Angry or negative thoughts shape angry or negative people. They do not result in patient, tolerant, compassionate beings. The same is true of our actions. War will never beget peace. Violence will never turn into kindness. The effects of our actions are consistent with their causes. And just like seeds, actions also take time to ripen.

A gardener cannot force a tree to bloom before its time. The seed will ripen according to its nature and in proportion to the nurturing it receives. Our bodies and minds are also like this. No matter how hard we push ourselves to run fast, our muscles cannot exceed their own capacity and development. Even if we strive to still our minds or will ourselves to be kinder, change will happen only when our consistent efforts ripen into their respective results, and not before.

Finally, as gardeners we are in charge of all the seeds in the storehouse—both those we choose to nurture and those we decide to ignore. If a tree is not growing the way we expected, it's not the seed's fault. The seed is not responsible if we have tilled the soil improperly, if we planted it in a hard bed of clay or forgot to water it. A neglected seed is definitely not another gardener's failure either.

Suppose our runner's partner asks him to accompany her to a party. Our friend agrees, and he stays up so late that night that in the morning he decides he's too tired to run. It's not his partner's fault that he didn't train that day, nor the fault of the people who threw the party. In fact, it's not a matter of finding fault at all. We all have to make choices, and when we understand that our actions are our responsibility, we're in a better position to choose wisely. As the Buddha said in a teaching called "The Five Remembrances," our actions are our true belongings. They are the only thing we "possess" in this life:

> I am of the nature to grow old. I cannot avoid growing old.
> I am of the nature to get sick. I cannot avoid sickness.
> I am of the nature to die. I cannot avoid death.
> All that is dear to me and everyone I love are of the nature
>   to change. I cannot avoid being separated from them.

My actions are my only true belongings. I cannot avoid the
consequences of my actions.
My actions are the ground upon which I stand.

Our actions are the seeds that will either bloom or wither away,
depending on the choices we make and the actions we take based
on those choices. So we could say that true discipline comes from
understanding that even casual choices and actions matter. Knowing that the seed of an action always matches its fruit, and that it
takes time to mature, then our task is to pick the right seeds to
water, and carefully and persistently choose actions that will help
those budding plants to grow. As with commitment, this requires a
certain degree of renunciation. We give up certain things in order
to devote our time and energy to others. Yet it's also important to
acknowledge the loss of those seeds that, based on the decisions
we've made, will not be able to grow to maturity in our lives.

During my late twenties, while at the monastery and well on
my way to monastic ordination, I had to grapple with the knowledge that, if I became a monk, I'd be unable to have children. I had
thought motherhood would be part of my path, yet when I arrived at
the monastery I felt that my calling lay there instead. So after much
reflection, I decided that I was more willing to live with the sadness
of not having children than with the sadness of not being a monk. I
made a choice, I watered that seed, and I spent some time mourning the seed I would not water. That is why I feel that, in order to
be whole, we need to recognize and allow the sadness or longing or
resentment we might feel at the sacrifices we make to support our
choices. The weightier the choices, the more we might have to sur-
render, so it's important to let ourselves grieve what can sometimes
be a significant loss. Otherwise we can end up feeling divided.

Who Is the True One?

Many years ago, in a small fishing village there lived a girl called
Senjo and a boy named Ochu. The two were cousins, and they were

so close and loved each other so dearly that all the villagers said each was like a sun to the other's moon.

"They will surely get married one day," they said. "They are made for each other." And when they heard this, Senjo and Ochu were overjoyed.

But as the two got older and the time came for Chokan, Senjo's father, to give away his only daughter in marriage, he decided that it would be best for her to wed a prosperous, more mature merchant called Hinryo instead. "He will be able to provide for you," he said to his daughter. "We will never lack for anything."

Ochu didn't believe that Chokan would go through with this plan, but Senjo knew her father. Once he made up his mind, there was nothing anyone could do to dissuade him. Still, she tried. She pleaded and begged and cried, but Chokan refused to budge. Finally Ochu understood that he was about to lose Senjo forever.

Late one night, Ochu packed a small canoe with some food and his few belongings. *I would rather never see Senjo again than see her married to another man*, he thought. He quietly slipped his boat into the water and set off downriver. As Ochu paddled, a full moon rose over the treetops, casting long shadows on the riverbank where crickets trilled in the reeds. After a while, he pulled in his paddle and lay on his back on the bottom of the boat staring up at the sky, his heart in pieces.

Suddenly, a loud rustling startled Ochu out of the half sleep he'd drifted into. Thinking he was about to be ambushed by robbers or a wild boar, he grabbed his wooden staff and prepared himself for an attack. He crouched low in the canoe and kept his gaze fixed on the riverbank. After a moment, a familiar figure burst out of the reeds into view of the drifting boat, where she was fully illuminated by the moon.

"Senjo!" Ochu yelled.

Quickly he paddled the canoe ashore. Senjo nimbly stepped into the boat and dropped her bundle next to Ochu's. The two held each other tightly.

"You're here," Ochu whispered in her ear.

Senjo nodded. "I'm here."

She sat facing Ochu and waited. Smiling, the young man picked up his paddle and began paddling with all his might, adding his strength to the current that was carrying them away from their village and toward the new life they would build together.

Years passed. Senjo gave birth to a boy and a girl, and a part of her felt she'd never been happier. But there was also a sadness in her that grew day by day. She missed her father and their village. She hadn't said goodbye, hadn't explained why she'd left. The more settled her life with Ochu became, the more she longed to return to their childhood home. After weeks of quiet struggle, Senjo called Ochu to her.

"Loving you, I left my home without Father's permission," she said, gently stroking her husband's face. "You have loved me too, and together we've made a wonderful life for ourselves. But the truth is, I miss Father more than I can bear. I long to see him and ask his forgiveness. He has grandchildren now, and he should meet them. It's time for us to go home."

Ochu nodded, relieved that Senjo had finally spoken. Through the years, he too had felt the weight of their leaving. He could see it reflected now and then in a gesture of Senjo's, in a look he caught when she thought he couldn't see. Chokan might not want to receive them, but they had to go back.

One clear summer morning, Senjo, Ochu, and their children waved to the neighbors gathered at the riverbank to send them off. They boarded the canoe and set off on their homeward journey. When after a few days they arrived at their old village, Senjo excitedly jumped out of the canoe, ready to run to her father. But Ochu held her back.

"Stay here with the children," he said. "You left your family because of me, so I should face your father first and ask his forgiveness."

Ochu tied the boat and slowly made his way to Senjo's old hut.

When he got to the top of the hill where a few huts were clustered, he saw old Chokan sitting outside on the ground, his back propped against a wall, his arms resting on his bent knees. The sun shone on his face and his eyes were closed.

The young man shyly called out to his uncle. Chokan opened his eyes and gazed at the visitor without recognizing him. Ochu walked forward slowly and greeted his uncle again.

"Ochu, it's you!" Chokan said, getting up stiffly to embrace his nephew. "I thought I'd never see you again."

Ochu lowered his eyes. "I'm sorry to have left as I did with Senjo, Uncle. I just couldn't bear to live without her. We built a home a few days' journey from here. We've come to ask your forgiveness and to rejoin the family, if you'll allow it."

"My daughter? What in heaven's name do you mean?" asked Chokan with a curious expression. "Senjo is right here. She took to her bed the night you left and has not gotten up since. She won't speak, she won't move. We've tried everything, but no potion, no prayer, no charm has been able to heal her."

"That can't be," Ochu shook his head. "Senjo has been with me all these years. She's down by the river right now with your grandchildren. They're all waiting to see you."

Chokan called to a boy who was passing by and asked him to check if visitors had come from upriver. The boy ran down to the water while the two men waited silently, each lost in his own thoughts. After a few minutes, the boy came back, panting.

"It's Senjo, Uncle," he said, sounding puzzled. "A boy and a girl are with her." The boy looked from one man to the other, but neither said anything. Chokan turned and went inside the hut. He approached the bed where his daughter lay with her eyes closed and leaned close to the pale face.

"Ochu is back, Senjo. He says you formed a family together. He says—" Chokan paused to swallow back his tears. "He's asking my forgiveness." Gently, he took his daughter's hand in his. "It's me who should ask for forgiveness, Senjo. I didn't understand how much you loved him. Now I know that your soul and your body were separated the day Ochu left."

Hearing this, Senjo opened her eyes, smiled, and spoke for the first time since she'd taken to her bed. "I never knew I was sick at home with you, Father. When I sensed that Ochu had left, I ran after his boat, feeling as if I were in a dream. I love him, and I love you. I am Ochu's wife and I am your daughter, but all this time, I didn't know who the true Senjo was."

With these words, Senjo got up from her bed and went outside. At the same time, the Senjo who had been waiting by the boat appeared at the top of the hill with her two children following close behind. When the two women saw one another, they smiled in recognition. Slowly, they walked toward each other until, in the presence of father and husband, they merged into one.

Many years later, Wuzu, an eleventh-century Zen master, turned this folk tale into a koan with a single question that Zen students would grapple with for the next thousand years. "Senjo and her soul were separated. Which is the true one?"

I ask you, which is the true Senjo? The one who stayed or the one who left? The one who returned or the one who woke up? Was Senjo the daughter and village member, or the mother and wife? What was Senjo's renunciation, and how was she made whole again?

If we're fortunate, discipline will teach us that, given how little we know of even those things that seem most certain, the most appropriate attitude to the mystery of a human life is humility. In the end, as powerful as discipline is, it is not invincibility. It doesn't soften our difficult choices or prevent us from hurting others in the process of choosing. But if we know how to wield it well, discipline can help clear out the clutter from our minds and lives so we can recognize what is most important to us and take the actions we need to protect it.

PRACTICE: STOP-START RUNNING
Practice focusing wholeheartedly on your breath.

A distracted, undisciplined mind is a mind lacking clarity and leaking energy. It is like a bucket with a hole or, to use a Buddhist simile, like a wild elephant. A concentrated mind, on the other hand, is stable and clear. It is a "firm post well sunk in the ground," as Soma Thera said. Having begun to develop our concentration in seated zazen, we will now take this discipline into running.

Before you begin, find a short route, something like a trail or a track. Choose familiar territory so you won't have to expend energy figuring out where you're going.

Run for ten or fifteen minutes at an easy pace to warm up. Then set a timer for ten minutes, thinking of this time as a period of running zazen. Just as with seated zazen, the focus of your moving meditation will be your breath. So as you run, pay attention to the sensation of the breath as it moves in and out of your body. Listen carefully to its sound, matching your stride to the inhalation and exhalation. Let all your awareness be filled with breath.

Continue running until you notice a thought that distracts you from the breath. Following the instruction for zazen, see the thought, let it go, and in this case, stop running. By this I don't mean you should slow down to a jog, but actually stop altogether. Take a moment to collect yourself, then start running again, placing all your attention back on the breath.

If you're honest with yourself, you'll most likely have to stop running every few steps, at least in the beginning. I realize this is annoying. But that is why this practice works. If you want to keep running, you really have to focus. So just remind yourself that you're not trying to get anywhere. The point of this practice is to train your mind to concentrate.

Continue running with your attention on your breath. See a thought. Let it go. Stop. Resume running. Do this over and over until the ten minutes are up, then let go of your breath and keep running at an easy pace. Allow your awareness to be open, stable, clear, and relaxed. If you want to repeat the practice, alternate between ten minutes of stop-start running and ten minutes of more open, relaxed movement. Finish with easy running. Afterward, note your observations in your journal.

Stop-start running is the first step in the development of concentration while running. Return to this practice often, for one of the central aspects of learning—and discipline—is repetition. So learn how to use your breath to anchor your attention while running. Let it be the firm post that keeps you grounded in your being.

5

Body

In college I had a yoga teacher who, in the middle of a particularly difficult pose, would turn to the class and say, "Where does this body begin? Where does it end?" Then, after a pause, she would add, "Find out."

What are the limits of this body? What is its origin and its nature? These are some of the questions that body practice seeks to address.

It is clear that my forty-six-year-old body is not the same body I occupied at five, twenty, or thirty-five. In many ways, I'm not the same person either. So where did those old selves go? Where will Zuisei go when this body dies?

The body is an excellent means for self-study because it's the aspect that we most readily identify as ourselves. Yet, for a culture utterly obsessed with the body, we are remarkably *dis*embodied. We love or hate our bodies. We primp and pump them, we nip and tuck them, we starve, stuff, neglect, or work them, but we rarely truly inhabit them. And we almost never ask ourselves, *Is this who I really am?*

In *The Interior Castle*, the great Spanish mystic Saint Teresa of Avila says, "We are incomparably more [foolish] when we do not strive to know who we are but limit ourselves to consider only roughly these bodies."

That is our loss—that we only *roughly* consider these bodies. We use them like vehicles to take us from one place to another without giving much thought to their nature, their function, or their relationship to mind.

Take your own body. You wouldn't say that your leg is you, would you? You would say it's a part of you, just as your feet are a part of you, your spleen, heart, skin. But when you look beyond these various elements, where or what is the essence of you? And how does the mind, which is formless, influence the body, which is made of form? This is such a basic question, but despite all of our scientific knowledge, we haven't yet come up with a satisfactory answer. The fact is, we simply don't know.

Right now, as I type this, I'm aware that I'm sitting at a wooden table next to the pool at my godparents' house. It is winter in Acapulco, so I'm wearing a light fleece over my T-shirt to ward off the predawn chill. My eyes can see hundreds of lights across the bay and in their glare, the quiet ripple of waves inching toward shore. I smell the ocean and next door, coffee and toast. Every now and then I have to bat away an eager mosquito dive-bombing my hands, and I marvel at the fact that they haven't yet found my bare ankles. My ears hear the rumble of trucks in the distance and closer by, a voice that is surprisingly insistent at this hour.

Because I sat here yesterday, I also know that in another half hour I'll be able to see bats zooming past and hear the crazy cackles of a flock of chachalacas holding court somewhere just out of sight. A handsome pair of *luis bienteveo* birds ("I see you well"), will stand by the side of the pool looking for worms in the well-cut lawn, their bright yellow chests and Zorro-like masks drawing the eye irresistibly.

My senses are taking in all of these stimuli, and my mind is quickly sorting through the information it's receiving to form a four-dimensional picture of reality, with me at its center. (That is the endless job of manas: to remind me that *I'm* the one who is experiencing all of this.) In addition, my brain is telling my fingers to type these words. Faithfully, my fingers obey, and as I write there is no break in the overall pattern.

It is an incredible process, if you think about it. Incredible that, moment to moment, I know I'm me, separate from the birds, the table, and the ocean, and that I can perform all sorts of tasks without losing sight of my surroundings. But there is more to this picture than what is evidenced by my senses. As Buddhism says, I'm not separate from all these various elements. Nothing is. Every component of this picture I call "reality" is arising simultaneously, which means that my mind, my body, and the phenomena I'm experiencing are all inseparable. If any of the three were missing, reality as I know it would not exist. Without a body, I could not perceive these sights and sounds and smells. Without a mind, I could not make sense of my perceptions, and reality would be just a jumble of unconnected stimuli. Without phenomena, there would be nothing to perceive. Consciousness, senses, and objects are all needed to form this perfect picture, which means that mind, body, and world are inextricably connected. Given this, what *is* the body? And how do we best study it in order to find out?

Still Running

At the end of one of my running retreats I was standing in the monastery's bookstore talking to a couple of the retreat participants. Overhearing our conversation, a man who was standing nearby approached us to discuss the benefits of teaching new runners about form and posture.

He said, "I've read a number of articles that argue that the best way for runners to learn good form is by running a lot. Formal instruction just gets in the way."

I was about to disagree when one of the women I'd been talking to spoke up.

"That works when you already know how to run. But for someone like me, learning good form at the beginning was very important. Not only did it help me to run faster, it also made it easier to pay attention to my body, which meant I was less likely to get injured or overtrain."

I added that it is like teaching people to do zazen. Beginners benefit from basic instruction, because when asked to sit on the floor, nine out of ten will sit slumped on top of the cushion with their legs crossed at the ankles and their knees in the air. Doing zazen like this for five or ten minutes will be uncomfortable, but trying to hold this posture without moving for half an hour or more will be excruciating. So it helps to learn a posture that will facilitate alertness and concentration. Yet within this basic form there is room for variation. Bodies differ, so differences in posture are normal and expected. Within limits, so are people's preferences. Some meditators like to sit low to the ground, using only the thinnest of cushions. Others need to sit on a higher seat. Some sit cross-legged on the floor, others prefer to kneel on a bench or sit in a chair.

Running is the same. We each have to account for our own mechanics and style, but following certain basic postural guidelines will ease both our running and our recovery. As my friend Colt demonstrated, there is a way to run that is natural, smooth, and effortless. Every part of our bodies moves as it should, in unison with every other part—like a seasoned orchestra whose musicians work seamlessly together to produce a harmonious sound.

"Besides," said the woman, "we teach technique in every other sport. I don't see why running should be an exception." Not to mention that running well feels good. Running badly doesn't. So even if you don't intend to run long distances and never want to compete in a race, knowing a few key principles will make your running safer, more enjoyable, and full of presence. This is the most important element of still running. The Buddha called it mindfulness. He said, when you're walking, know that you're walking. When standing, know that you're standing. When sitting, know that you're sitting. But this is not how most of us use our minds.

Multitasking is the favorite mode of our harried and efficiency-focused culture, even though it is actually an extremely inefficient way to use our attention. Although it appears as if we're capable of simultaneously holding several things in mind, this is an illusion. Our brains can focus on only one stimulus at a time, so "multitasking" is really a lightning-speed shuffling of attention from one object to another, a process that psychologists call "context shifting."

If you're watching a movie while having dinner, for example, your brain is constantly shifting context from a bite of pizza to a movie frame or two, back to the taste of melted cheese in your mouth, and again to the story on-screen. Back and forth you move from one to the other, losing a little more focus every time you shift. Is it any wonder we often feel so depleted?

The practice of running zazen requires that we deliberately slow down and let our attention work as it is really meant to: undividedly. That is why I call this kind of running *still running*. It is running that is grounded, focused, and effortless—the kind of running you can disappear into by letting your body and mind dissolve into movement, into breath.

The teachings I've offered so far on practice, intent, commitment, and discipline, as well as the ones that follow on body, mind, effort, stillness, and movement, are all for the purpose of developing this new way of moving. Let me warn you, however, that if you dread the act of running or if you're used to distracting yourself while doing it, at first you may resist this practice. If you've become accustomed to running while listening to music, watching television, or reading a magazine, running with complete awareness will feel challenging because you'll have to face your boredom, discomfort, or resistance. But if you can stay present and patient through the initial struggle, you'll find that the energy and quiet of still running builds over time and with practice, can also translate to other activities.

So as you develop your running practice, learn to keep your mind focused and your body relaxed. How? By paying attention to your movement at a very basic level. By acknowledging, first of all, the miracle that it is to be able to run at all.

The Miracle of a Human Body

In the 1980s an artificial intelligence researcher by the name of Hans Moravec said that, while it's relatively easy to program computers to do high-level tasks like math and chess, it is virtually impossible for them to imitate low-level activities, like the walking of a toddler. The reason behind this paradox—which became known as Moravec's Paradox—is that sensory-motor and largely unconscious skills such as walking have evolved over the past several million years. Reasoning and intelligence, on the other hand, are only a few thousand years old and are therefore easier to replicate. The implication is clear: it has taken us millions of years to learn how to walk effortlessly.

It's a shame we don't remember our tenuous first steps, the effort required just to keep ourselves upright. A shame we've forgotten the all-consuming task of learning to place one foot before the other. Because, as a Chinese proverb says, "The miracle is not to fly in the air nor to walk on water, but to walk on the earth."

I sometimes do forget what a wonder it is that I have a healthy, working body. But putting on my running shoes and heading outside will quickly remind me of the gift I've been given, as well as the responsibility I have to care for it. It is my responsibility to strengthen, feed, and rest my body, and to make use of it as well as I can. This means knowing it intimately and paying attention to the signals that tell me when something is not working smoothly. So consider using the following guidelines to either establish or refine your form. Think of them as the scaffolding for a strong, focused, and relaxed running practice.

Begin by standing with your feet hip-width apart, your shoulders relaxed, and your arms resting loosely at your sides. If you can, work with a partner or stand in front of a full-length mirror.

Place your attention on the crown of your head and press it up toward the ceiling, then relax your shoulders again. Look at your reflection, or have your partner give you feedback. Are your shoulders level? Are they squared and relaxed? One of your shoulders may be higher than the other. This is common, but working with your posture will help you become aware and therefore not exacerbate the imbalance.

Now look down at your feet without bending over. Can you see them? If you can't, your hips are probably too far forward. If you have lower back pain when you run, this is a sign that you're leading with your hips. To correct this, move your hips back with your hands until they're directly under your shoulders. Level your pelvis by engaging the lower abdomen and slightly tuck in the tailbone. Be careful not to tighten your glutes as you do this.

Place one hand on your chest, the other on your belly. Lengthen the back of your neck. Look at your feet again. If you can see them, lift your head and close your eyes. Try to memorize this posture. Keep retraining yourself to stand with your hips and shoulders aligned, your abdominals lightly engaged, and the back of your neck long.

Turn sideways to the mirror or your partner, and study your posture again. Is your head directly over your spine? If it isn't, tuck in your chin slightly. Pay attention to your jaw: is it clenched or relaxed? As you run, you want to keep your mouth, jaw, and throat soft. Bend your knees slightly.

Whether I'm running on the road or a treadmill, I always practice keeping my center of gravity low and my knees slightly bent so my legs can turn smoothly under me. I want all of my momentum to propel me forward instead of up and down, where the energy will dissipate.

Turn again to face the mirror or your partner. Bend your elbows ninety degrees so your forearms are parallel to the ground. Swing your arms as if you are running, and notice if your hands are crossing the midline of your body (imagine a line running down from your nose to the navel, separating the right and left sides of the body). Be careful not to waste valuable forward motion by letting your hands swing too far across your chest. Concentrate on easily moving your arms so your elbows and fists are alternately aligning with your torso. Your hands should be relaxed, held in a gentle fist, with your thumbs resting on your bent fingers. Don't twist your wrists or pump your arms as you swing.

Relax your arms, and try leaning forward slightly from your ankles while keeping your torso straight. To do this, you'll once again have to engage your abdomen and press up through the crown of the head. Don't fold at the waist. If you're working with a partner, stand facing one another about three feet apart, bend your elbows, and interlock hands for support. Now lean toward your partner by letting yourself "fall" forward. Don't forget to keep your spine long and your abdomen engaged. There should be a straight line from your head all the way down to your feet. Leaning from the ankles keeps your feet directly under or slightly behind you as you run. Instead of reaching forward, you'll let your stride open up behind you.

Stand up straight again, and practice picking up your heel so that it clears the ankle of the opposite foot as you take a step. Focus on the *lift* of the foot, rather than its downward movement. Think of a horse prancing. The lighter your stride, the less impact on your knees.

There is quite a bit of talk in the running world about the best kind of foot strike: heel, midfoot, or forefoot. In general, mid- and forefoot strikes are considered biomechanically sounder, while heel striking is thought to channel a lot more pressure to the joints. One analogy I read likened a heel strike to smashing your fist into a wall. Practice picking up your foot (not your knee) with each step and letting it float forward as you touch the ground lightly at the front or middle of the foot.

In high school one of my favorite workouts was doing sprints wearing a weight belt with a car tire attached to it. My teammates and I would do several repetitions of 20- or 30-foot sprints—the most ambitious of us with another runner sitting on the tire. Then we'd remove the belt and do a few more sprints. It was exhilarating to suddenly feel so weightless. Years later I had a similar feeling when I switched from a heel to a forefoot strike. It was as if an invisible weight had been lifted off my back—suddenly I could run lightly and fast.

Another important element in the development of your running form is gait. The three main gaits are pronation, overpronation, and supination. Pronation is the natural rolling in of the foot to absorb shock and distribute weight evenly during each step.

If you have a pair of old running shoes, take note of their wear marks, for this will help you identify your gait and the kind of shoe you should use to minimize injuries. Pronation, the ideal gait, causes a shoe to wear out evenly across the forefoot. Overpronating makes the feet tilt inward, wearing out the inner edge of the heel and front of the sole under the ball of the foot. Supinating wears out the outer edge of the shoe as the foot rolls out. Various kinds of running shoes have been designed to correct for these imbalances by providing additional cushioning or stability. If you're not sure which shoe is best suited to your gait, consult a specialist. Many running stores are staffed with experienced runners who can help you identify your gait and the shoe most appropriate for it. When you find a shoe that works, consider buying at least a second pair. Rotating two pairs of shoes will make them last longer, and you won't have to go through the same trial and error when your shoe is replaced by a newer—but not necessarily better—model.

Finally, there is the question of stretching. As with everything else in running, there are many different opinions about whether stretching is good or even necessary. Personally, I never do static stretches before running—only the joint exercises I describe in the practice that follows. But I always take the time to stretch afterward. A quick Internet search will yield a number of stretching routines for runners, and I highly recommend you follow one or more of them. Doing even a few minutes of post-run stretching can help to prevent injuries as well as ease your next day's run.

Following these posture guidelines, your runs should feel smoother and less effortful. But remember that they are only that—guidelines—and many successful runners flout them outright. Paula Radcliffe, who in 2003 set the women's world record for the marathon and has run four out of the five fastest times in the history of the women's race, runs ramrod straight, reaches forward with her feet, and overpronates, which causes her toes to splay outward. She also swings her arms across her body, and she leaps so high with each step it could be said that she bounds rather than runs. Saif Saaeed Shaheen, a 3,000-meter steeplechase champion, also flails his arms and almost leans back as he runs. Many experienced marathon runners are heel strikers. All of which goes to show that, in the end, each one of us has to work with our particular body.

So if these guidelines help, use them. If not, throw them away and find ones that do. I've always thought of zazen as the practice of unburdening yourself. Running zazen can be the same. If you allow both disciplines to inform one another, then your running—and your life—can be joyful and light.

PRACTICE: YOUR RUNNING FORM
Develop a good running form.

Before you go out for your next run, take five or ten minutes to stretch your joints, starting with your ankles. First, lift one foot and turn it in circles—eight repetitions clockwise, then eight counterclockwise. Repeat with the other foot. Then place your hands on your knees and draw circles with both knees, eight times in each direction. Do the same with your hips, your arms, and your head.

Still standing, separate your feet about three or four feet apart and place your hands on the back of your head. From the waist, pivot slowly to the right, letting your torso turn like a corkscrew—first your hips, then your lower, middle, and upper back. Turn your neck, reaching as far around as you can go. Return to center by reversing this sequence, then pivot to the left and repeat. Return to center again.

Next place your hands on your hips, and on an inhale lift your chin, tilt your head back, and look up. With the exhale, bend forward at the waist. Lead with your chin so your back remains long and straight. Once you've bent as far down as you can go, relax your head and look down or, if you have folded over completely, between your legs. Do this a couple of times, coming up with the inhale leading with your chin and bending on the exhale relaxing your head. Shake out your arms and legs. Now you're ready to start running.

Begin by jogging slowly, letting your body warm up. After about ten minutes, choose one area of your body on which to focus for the next ten minutes. This will be the anchor for your attention, just as breath was your anchor in the practice of Stop-Start Running (page 46).

If you tend to drag your feet, commit to focusing on the action of lifting your ankles by stepping lightly without lifting the knees too much. Focus on the lift rather than the strike of your foot, but don't push off with your toes. Keep your whole foot relaxed, and listen to your steps. Do you hear a slapping, skidding, or thudding sound? This means you're not stepping lightly. See if you can make your stride quiet and light.

Alternatively, focus on keeping your pelvis level by engaging the abdominal muscles and lightly tucking in the sacrum without tightening your glutes. Or concentrate on leaning from your ankles, or running with slightly bent knees, or swinging your arms easily. Whatever posture guideline you decide to focus on, keep your attention on it for the full ten minutes. When the time is up, relax your focus and run easily for another ten minutes, then choose the same guideline and focus on it for another ten minutes. Alternate between focusing and relaxing, but avoid switching from one guideline to another during the same run. It takes time to learn each of them, and in order to develop your concentration you'll have to work through the restlessness that comes from focusing on a single object over a period of time.

Most of us have a rather loose definition of focus. We are so used to certain movements, certain patterns of mind, that we don't even notice that we're not truly present. Yet single-minded focus is just that: single-minded. When running, allow your awareness to rest completely on the lift of the ankle, the contact of your foot on the ground, the swing of your arms. Undoubtedly, this degree of concentration takes effort. But as we've seen, the more we practice staying focused, the easier it becomes. Focus begets focus. So when you start to get distracted, remind yourself that you are learning to use your body in order to realize the nature of that very body.

As my yoga teacher would ask, where does this body begin? Where does it end? A human life is long enough to seek an answer, but it's too short not to ask, so don't wait to find out.

6

Effort

A young monk named Sona was practicing meditation one morning in the Cool Wood near Rajagaha on Vulture Peak Mountain. He was young and earnest, and when he wasn't sitting in meditation, he was walking on a short trail leading from his hut to a small clearing in the woods. To and fro he paced for hours, until the soles of his feet were bleeding. Finally, tired and sore, Sona sat down on a fallen log to rest.

"I'm persistent, yet my mind is still restless and full of clinging," he found himself thinking. "What if I abandoned the monastic life and rejoined my family? There are other ways to make merit besides practicing meditation."

You can see the wheels turning in Sona's mind as he constructs his argument: If he goes back to lay life, he can make merit by building stupas and giving alms to the mendicant monks. He'll be able to attend services and maybe even do a little meditation, but most of his time will be dedicated to work and family. His parents will be delighted to have him back, and since there are many other monks in the *sangha*, he won't be missed. And why does the wandering life have to be so hard, anyway?

Who hasn't faced doubt like this at some point in their lives? *Why in the world am I doing this?* we ask ourselves. This job, this relationship, this sport, this art. *What if I quit while I still can? After all, there are other ways to do good work.*

This moment of doubt is pivotal. It's the moment when our commitment either holds or breaks. Maybe our intent has shifted, which means our commitment needs to shift with it. Such a moment requires clear discernment, which is sometimes difficult to access on our own. Fortunately for Sona, the Buddha was staying near the Cool Wood, also practicing meditation. He read the young monk's mind and instantly appeared in the clearing where Sona was resting. (In many stories written after the Buddha's death he is said to have had both omniscience and supernatural powers.)

After taking a seat and folding his legs under him in the meditation posture, the Buddha turned to the young monk and asked, "My friend, weren't you just thinking of leaving the community and returning to your family so you could enjoy a life of wealth and comfort?"

Cornered, Sona had no choice but to answer truthfully. "Yes, Lord. I was."

"Mmmh," said the Buddha. "Tell me, didn't you used to play the lute?"

"Yes, I did," said Sona.

"Venerable Sona, what do you think? When stringing your lute, what happened if the strings were too tight?"

Sona answered, "They would break."

"And if they were too loose?"

"My lute wouldn't play."

The Buddha nodded. "What about when the strings were neither too tight nor too loose, but were tuned to be right on pitch?"

"I was able to play, Lord," said Sona, his face relaxing as he understood the Buddha's meaning.

The Buddha smiled gently. "In the same way, Sona, too much zeal leads to restlessness, too little persistence leads to laziness. Thus you should determine the right pitch for your persistence, attune the pitch of the five faculties, and there pick up your theme."

Determine the right pitch for your persistence. What do you want? How much do you want it? What are you willing to do to achieve it? What kind of effort are you willing to exert? It certainly can't be mindless effort. It cannot be blind. It must be pitched to the five faculties of sight, hearing, smell, taste, and touch. It must also match your theme. In other words, commitment, discipline, and effort must all match your intent. And in order to be effective, your effort must be skillful, and it must be right.

Right Effort

Right effort is the sixth factor in the Noble Eightfold Path, the Buddha's teaching on the means to self-liberation.

"All of my teaching can be encapsulated in a single sentence," the Buddha said. "I teach suffering and its cessation."

Elaborating, he then offered the Four Noble Truths. The First Noble Truth says that life is suffering. All of life is suffering, because we constantly want what we don't have, reject what we have, and lose what we want and have. No matter who we are or how much we own, every single one of us experiences these three types of suffering. The Second Noble Truth says that the cause of this suffering is craving— our desire to hold on to pleasure and avoid pain. But there is a way to relieve suffering, states the Third Noble Truth. The Fourth Noble Truth shows how to do this: by means of the Noble Eightfold Path, made up of right view, right thought, right speech, right action, right livelihood, right effort, right mindfulness, and right concentration.

A number of excellent books have dealt extensively with the Eightfold Path. So for our purposes, I'll focus only on the last three factors of the path and their relationship to stillness and movement, meditation and activity.

Traditionally, *right effort* is understood as the "correct" or "appropriate" focus necessary to identify and cultivate skillful or beneficial actions and to prevent or stop unskillful ones. Used more broadly, it is also energy that is skillful and relevant to whatever task we've set for ourselves. To continue the musical analogy, it's effort that is appropriate in pitch, volume, and timbre. It allows us to work in concert with, rather than against, ourselves by helping us to identify those thoughts and actions that sustain the melody we've chosen while also letting go of the noise that interferes with its harmony.

"Singing is the defiance of air loss," a voice teacher once said to me. "As singers we expect to be as capable—as consistent and energetic—at the beginning of a note as at its end. This is ridiculous. And yet, that's what singing is—sustaining a note with intensity all the way to the end." Then she explained that, in order to do this, we must learn to allow the right amount of breath to move through our vocal cords. Too little breath, and the sound is limp. Too much, and our pitch wavers or our breath runs out. We have to use just the right amount to produce a clear, sustained note.

The challenge, of course, is to know how much and what kind of effort is right, not just for singing but for any activity. When it comes to running, how do we know when we need to challenge ourselves and when we should relax? How do we refine our discipline without becoming inflexible? When do we take others' advice, and when do we trust ourselves?

The late Harriet Thompson was a marathon runner and classical pianist who in 2015 ran a marathon in seven hours, seven minutes, and forty-two seconds, still the fastest time in her category (she was ninety-two). Thompson started running long distances in her seventies in order to raise money for leukemia and lymphoma research. Soon after she completed her sixteenth marathon, a reporter asked her how she felt about her performance. She answered she was happy—she'd once again come in first in her age group—but also sorry she hadn't been able to train more because she'd been struggling with a staph infection in her leg, the result of treatment she had received for squamous cell carcinoma.

I wouldn't be surprised if more than one person tried to dissuade Thompson from running. "Aren't you too old to be doing this?" "What about your cancer?" "Don't you need to rest?" "What if you hurt your knees/your back/your hips?" But regardless of what drove her, my guess is that Thompson ran because she had to. Because it kept her alive and vibrant in ways that only she could understand.

On the other hand, an athlete like Tatyana McFadden would not have questioned Thompson for an instant. The Russian-born American Paralympian was born with spina bifida, a condition that left her paralyzed from the waist down. Shortly after her birth, McFadden's mother abandoned her in an orphanage. McFadden's guardians were unable to afford a wheelchair, so she walked on her hands for the first six years of her life. At eight, she began competing in wheelchair races, and in the two decades that followed, she proceeded to rack up an impressive number of medals. By 2013 she had become the first person of any gender or ability to win four major world marathons in the same year. McFadden has since been called the greatest wheelchair athlete in the world.

Whenever I'm feeling uninspired, I think of Thompson or McFadden, just two of the athletes who have refused to let themselves be bound by other's expectations, and instead set and followed their own.

Right effort requires a profound level of trust. It asks that we be fully aware of our limits and also that we be courageous enough to go beyond them. But in order to do this, each one of us must first determine the right amount of energy to respond to our circumstances.

Just the Right Amount

In Zen there is a formal meal ceremony called *oryoki*, Japanese for "the container that holds the right amount to respond to a need." The term refers to the traditional monastic begging bowl, but it can also apply to each of us: we are containers with just the right amount of energy and ability to respond to various needs.

During the two decades that I lived at Zen Mountain Monastery, I followed a rigorous daily schedule. Five days on, two days off,

I was up around three thirty in the morning, in bed at nine thirty at night. Almost every hour of my day was scheduled and spent working, studying, and doing zazen in the company of others. In short, it was not a way of life that allowed for much downtime.

Shortly after arriving there, I realized I had two choices: I could power through the days hoping that my energy would carry me, or I could learn to use my energy well. I knew how to work until collapse; I had done that repeatedly throughout my life. But I also understood I couldn't sustain that way of being forever. So when I learned about right effort, I knew I needed to take it up as a practice. I needed to become a student of energy and fatigue, of rest, balance, and recovery.

One afternoon during that time I was reading Charles Frazier's novel *Cold Mountain* when a passage leapt out at me. Ada Monroe, a city-bred young woman who, by her own admission, can quote Homer but doesn't know how to do anything useful, has been given two tasks: to burn the brush from a field and to split a black oak. Ruby, her neighbor and helper, is a feral woman who can kill chickens with her bare hands and will not back down from any task. Yet both women are slight, and Ada worriedly asks if they're really fit for that kind of labor. "It doesn't necessarily require pure power," Ruby says in response. "Just pacing, patience, rhythm . . ." The main thing, she explains, is to not get ahead of yourself. It's to move at a rhythm that you can sustain—to do as much as you can and still be able to get up and begin again the next day. No more and no less.

That's it, I thought. *That's what I need to find—a rhythm I can sustain.* So far my effort had been too strenuous, too uneven. I decided then and there that I would practice oryoki, not just while eating but in everything I did.

As I began to explore what it really means to exert the right amount of effort, I noticed two things. First, I didn't really know how to rest. I rushed from one activity to the next compelled by my anxiety to get things done and rarely gave myself the time and space to do anything fully. Second, I used too much energy to accomplish even the simplest of tasks. It was as if I'd only been equipped with an on-off switch and had no way to modulate my effort or pace. I understood that, by preference and temperament, I was energetic, but I knew from experience that that energy could become manic if I wasn't careful. And if I was honest with myself, I would also say that I often hid in my hard work and the feeling of accomplishment it gave me. It was easier to labor than to feel. Yet Zen practice demanded that I slow down and investigate what I was doing and why. It required that I stop and actually be with myself. But I didn't yet know how to contain the energy that came from strong concentration, so I sometimes felt even more wired after zazen. All of these factors contributed to energy swings, but I could sense there was something else—something I needed to understand more clearly. Eventually I saw it as the subtle connection between effort, mindfulness, and concentration.

Right effort, right mindfulness, and right concentration are grouped together in the Noble Eightfold Path under the category of concentration, or *samadhi*: single-pointedness of mind. In one sense we could say that right effort *is* mindfulness and concentration. Concentration is the ability to focus the mind, to direct our attention and keep it stable. Mindfulness is seeing *what* is arising as we concentrate. Paired with concentration and mindfulness, right effort is the discernment of the quality and quantity of energy needed to match any given activity.

No one would argue that chopping and stacking a cord of wood requires a different kind of energy than creating a stained-glass window. Writing a book requires a certain kind of effort; so does developing a piece of software or offering counseling to someone in distress. Practicing right effort means allowing our minds and bodies to quiet down so we can let each activity teach us the kind of focus and energy it requires. Instead of doing *to*, we do *with*. We learn when to press and when to relax. When to focus narrowly and when to hold the big picture in mind. With practice our effort gradually becomes effortless until we can merge with the task at hand. This is when skill becomes mastery—the perfect fusion of body, mind, and action.

The Right Pitch for Your Persistence

"Have I ever told you about the windsurfer?" my father said. We were sitting at the dining room table, eating peanuts and talking. "This happened several years ago. I'm surprised I never told you the story."

One summer, said my father, he, his partner, and a friend were having drinks at a seaside restaurant while they waited for another friend to arrive so they could all go to a wedding. "It was a beautiful, clear afternoon," my father said, smiling as he remembered the day. "There was a light breeze, and the sun was beginning to set. I was sitting quietly, just looking at the ocean while the women talked, when at a distance I spotted a windsurfer—just the silhouette of the sail against the sky. I watched for a while, and when the figure got closer I could see it was a woman. She was very good. She was maneuvering that sail as if it were weightless."

My father nodded approvingly. He's a sailor and had recognized mastery when he saw it.

"But that's not all," he added, taking a sip of his Coke. "When she got closer to shore I could see she was wearing a dress—a sequined gown that came just below her knee."

"A sequined gown?" I repeated dumbly.

My father nodded. "And high heels." He paused. "She was surfing in full evening wear. I watched her maneuver her board ashore and slide off it effortlessly onto the soft sand, heels and all. She came up to us smiling and glittering. As it turns out, she was the friend we were waiting for."

My father drank the last of his Coke and set the empty glass on the table.

"And by the way, she was also a pretty good dancer."

Whether we are running, windsurfing, painting a canvas, or

playing the violin, finding the right pitch for our persistence allows us to disappear into what we're doing. It allows us to drop our self-consciousness so we can give ourselves over to the melody we've chosen and let it show us how it should be played.

So listen carefully to each note of your theme. Be patient and persistent, for anything worth doing takes time. Yet know that, when the lute strings are pitched just right, the playing will be effortless. Lute and player disappear, and all that is left is the melody itself, clear and true.

PRACTICE: RHYTHM AND CADENCE

Establish your running cadence.

In this practice you'll work on finding the pitch of your persistence while running. This is your rhythm or cadence.

Make sure you have a watch or timer with you when you go out on your next run. And if you have a metronome—either on your phone or watch—that's even better. Alternatively, you can use a regular timer and train yourself to maintain a steady rhythm by counting your steps for short periods throughout your run.

Take the first ten minutes to warm up by running at a slow, relaxed pace. Keep in mind the posture guidelines, and notice if there are any areas in your body that are tight or that need particular attention. If your mind is sluggish, anchor your awareness in your breath. Remember to keep your stride light.

Part of the practice of still running is identifying what you need to focus on. As I begin my daily run, I always do a quick mind and body scan to check how I'm feeling and to determine what kind of work I need to do that day. I ask myself whether I need to sharpen my focus by concentrating on my breath or posture, or whether I keep my mind open and relaxed. Should I generate energy by pushing myself a little or take it slow but steady? Over time, I've learned to read my body's signals so I can respond to them appropriately. This is how I determine the pitch of my persistence, the right amount of effort needed for that particular run.

After you've run easily for ten minutes, work your way up toward your usual speed. Then, focusing on one foot—let's say the right—count the number of times it strikes the ground in a minute. Do this a couple of times to make sure you have the right count. The number will be somewhere between sixty and ninety steps, depending on your speed and form. Now multiply the result by two. This is your cadence, or tempo—the rate at which your legs turn under you as you run.

Recreational runners have cadences between 140 and 170 steps per minute. Elite runners are closer to 180. If your cadence is less than 140, you can train yourself to run faster and with better form by focusing on gradually increasing the number of steps you take per minute.

Having a higher cadence is important because it prevents you from overstriding or bouncing, both of which waste energy and create more impact on your knees. Shorter steps and a quicker cadence keep your feet under rather than in front of you, making for a smoother, lighter stride. I also find that maintaining a steady cadence throughout my run encourages a kind of stillness in my movement, a "space" in which my mind and body can rest within that stable, rhythmic stride.

Even when running outside, imagine you're on a treadmill whose belt is moving smoothly under you. Don't forget to keep your knees slightly bent and your body leaning from your ankles. As you start to run faster, allow your stride to open up *behind* you, not in front.

To stay focused and to ensure you're running with good form, count your steps every three minutes, then every five, then every ten, testing that you've maintained the same cadence throughout. If you're running well, your steps should feel steady and light, your breath even, your mind quiet. Otherwise, slow down a bit. Is your cadence too high to maintain throughout a full run? Take it down a few steps per minute and gauge the effect.

When you have five or ten minutes left in your run, let go of checking your cadence and just run. Go as fast or as slow as you want. Relish the feel of your body moving through space.

When you're done, take some time to cool down and stretch.

Keep working on finding a rhythm that you can sustain over time, in all aspects of your life. Notice when you're pushing too much or when you're going slack. Identify whether the sluggishness is in your body or in your mind, and find ways to inspire yourself to do what you say you want to do. Attune the pitch of your persistence to your five senses—and to the sixth sense, mind—so you can learn what it means to do neither too much nor too little, to respond with just the right amount of concentration, mindfulness, and effort to the need at hand.

7

Breath

On a cool spring morning, a Zen teacher and his student are going for a walk. The last traces of snow have melted from the ground, and tiny buds are beginning to show on the tips of the cherry branches. Bundled in their robes, master and disciple walk easily as the day slowly grows warmer. Their walk leads nowhere in particular. They are walking simply to walk, while all around them birds chirp quietly as if trying on their voices for the day.

After a while, the two men come upon a stream. The teacher sits down on the grassy bank with his back against the trunk of an alder. Like a puppy, the student plops himself on the ground, his legs crossed under him. His every movement says he's eager to impress the master. Quiet on the walk, he now prattles on about this and that teaching, peppering his own thoughts with bits of relevant commentaries. Every now and then he sneaks a glance at his teacher, checking his expression. The older man just listens, his eyes half-closed against the glare of the sun reflecting off the water.

"How is your zazen practice?" the teacher asks when the student finally grows still.

"Oh, you know," says the young man without looking at his teacher. In his mouth is a young grass shoot and he is relishing the bitter, lemony taste. "The breath is so boring."

Like a flash, the teacher throws himself on his student and with one quick move, rolls the younger man's upper body into the stream. He places one strong hand between his student's shoulder blades, the other on the back of his head, and pushes down hard to hold him underwater. Caught off guard, at first the student freezes. Then, when he realizes his teacher will not let go, he begins struggling. He tries to reach back to grab the older man's robe, but immediately his arm is pinned down under the teacher's leg. Desperate now, the young man tries to get purchase on the grass to wriggle out from under the teacher's grasp, but he can barely move. Another long moment passes before the teacher yanks him out of the water by pulling on his collar. Completely drenched, the student sits on the grass coughing and gasping for breath as the teacher looks at him searchingly.

"Still boring?" he asks.

The Four Foundations of Mindfulness

Boredom thrives on inattention. We take, on average, twenty thousand breaths a day. Our lives literally depend on this most basic function, yet we are usually unaware that it's happening. The breath is the vehicle of our life force; without breath, we cannot live. And without attention to our breath, we live half-consciously. That is why so many contemplative practices use the breath as the primary object of meditation.

In the *Satipatthana Sutta* (The Discourse on the Four Foundations of Mindfulness), the Buddha describes a practitioner who, sitting down quietly to contemplate her breath, is aware of it in this way:

Mindful, she breathes in and mindful, she breathes out.
Thinking, "I breathe in long," she understands when she is
    breathing in long.
Thinking, "I breathe out long," she understands when she
    is breathing out long.

Thinking, "I breathe in short," she understands when she
is breathing in short.

Thinking, "I breathe out short," she understands when she
is breathing out short.

Notice that the Buddha doesn't say the practitioner needs to control her breath. He doesn't say she should breathe long, deep, even breaths. He says she's mindful of the breath just as it is. Being mindful, she notices when her breath is long or short. Being mindful, she sees when she's breathing fully and when she's not. She knows when her breath is ragged and shallow, filled with tension and anxiety, or deep and even, quiet and relaxed.

The Buddha considered the breath the most important object of meditation—the gateway to enlightenment. Even after decades of practice, he periodically took time away from his sangha to go on solitary retreat in order to practice *anapanasati*, "mindfulness of breathing."

Mindfulness, or *sati*, is the ability to remember or to keep an object in mind. As I mentioned before, it is also the ability to see the object we are concentrating on: the breath, a thought, a feeling. *Right mindfulness* is made up of what in Buddhism are called the Four Foundations of Mindfulness: mindfulness of the body (especially of the breath), of feelings, of mind, and of thoughts or mental formations. To study these foundations, a practitioner uses mindfulness, alertness, and resolve, all of which rely on appropriate attention. "Appropriate" here specifically means attention that gives us insight into the problem of suffering and its alleviation and more broadly, attention that matches the object of our meditation. This is important because it is possible to be concentrated yet mindless. It is possible to be very focused and not see the object we're focusing on at all.

Halfway through my first weeklong *sesshin*, or silent meditation retreat, I was assigned to work in the monastery garden. The gardener was an old British nun with a singsong voice and a throat-clearing habit—a nervous little squeak with which she prefaced every sentence, as if she were unsure whether she should be speaking at all.

She walked me over to one of the raised garden beds and asked me to weed it. I suppose I looked like an outdoor type, because she didn't check whether I'd ever tended a garden. I hadn't. *But how hard can it be?* I thought, and plunged my hands into the dirt with relish.

It was July, and already warm though it was only eight thirty in the morning. My sleeves rolled up to my shoulders, I crouched next to the bed and began to pull weeds as fast as I could, determined to show the old nun that no one could work faster than I could. I had been doing zazen for three days, so my mind felt relatively quiet, but I was also buzzing with energy. I worked quickly—feverishly, really—without giving much thought to what I was doing.

At one point, a voice in my head interrupted my trance. *These weeds are growing awfully straight.* I felt a quick tightening of my stomach, a warning sign that I chose to ignore. I was doing too well to stop, I thought, so like an ox I lowered my head and kept going.

At the end of an hour and a half, when the work period was over, I proudly called over the nun to show her my work. She took one look at the bed and quickly walked away, muttering to herself. Confused, I stood where I was and waited. On the other side of the garden now, the nun stood a couple of feet from the fence, her back to me. She looked up at the sky, then down at the stones under her feet. She shook her head, shrugged her shoulders, then came back to where I was standing.

"You pulled a whole bed of carrots," she said, her voice rising past singsong into a cry.

It was a long time before I was assigned to the garden again.

Unfortunately, this kind of mindlessness is common. In our attempt to concentrate, we stop thinking or discerning. This is not what the Buddha had in mind, of course, when he spoke of single-pointed attention. Pulling carrots for weeds is one thing, yet every day there are a thousand ways in which we miss what's right before our eyes. Almost invariably, the result is more suffering for us and those around us.

Think of a morning when you woke up with a vague feeling of discomfort. Maybe you had a bad dream. Maybe you ate something that upset your stomach and now you're feeling off. Maybe you're processing an emotion you're not even aware of. Not being aware, you walk around feeling out of sorts. But you don't like this, so you are also unconsciously looking for an emotional release. Looking, you will find. The stack of bills your partner has left on the dining room table, your son's muddy boots by the door, your roommate's makeup on the dresser—these are all perfect excuses to start a fight. Before you even know what's happening, you're yelling, dredging up every instance of carelessness the other person has shown during the past ten years. If you're lucky, they'll know to walk away and not engage again until you've come to your senses. If you're not, they'll join the shouting match.

A consistent zazen practice helps us to quiet the noise of our minds through the development of concentration, and mindfulness helps us to pay attention to our experience in a very basic, unfiltered way. In the example above, mindfulness helps us to first realize *that* we're feeling something. The next step is to discern *what* we're feeling and *how* to respond to it skillfully instead of reactively.

In the *Sedaka Sutta*, the Buddha teaches his monks about mindfulness by giving them the following metaphor. Imagine a man, he says, who craves pleasure and avoids pain, who wants to live and does not want to die. Now imagine this man has been charged with carrying on his head a bowl filled to the brim with oil that he must deliver to a beauty queen who is singing and dancing in front of a throng of adoring fans. Carefully the man must walk through the crowd without spilling a single drop, for if he does, a swordsman walking behind him will chop off his head.

"What do you think, friends?" says the Buddha to his monks. "Will this man let himself be distracted?"

"No, of course not," they say.

"Well," he says, "the bowl of oil is mindfulness. This is how you should train yourselves in mindfulness of the body. Give mindfulness the reins, and take it as your ground; steady it, consolidate it, and undertake it well."

Taking mindfulness as our ground means remembering to pay attention moment to moment. It means remaining alert and resolute in our desire to be awake and present to our lives. Why? Because as this unusual sutra points out, our lives actually do depend on it.

Reclaiming Our Lives

Years ago, I watched a gymnast perform a complicated routine on a balance beam at a circus. Two burly twins were carrying the beam on their shoulders, and every time the gymnast did a flip or a jump, they shifted the beam slightly in order to catch her.

After a particularly harrowing move, it occurred to me that, given the gymnast's line of business, she couldn't afford to not be present. A momentary slip of focus, a split-second wavering of attention, and she'd break an arm or worse. And although her act was short—seven or eight minutes at most—she repeated it in exactly the same way day after day, sometimes twice a day, for weeks on end. Like the man with the bowl of oil on his head, her life depended on her ability to remain mindful.

Abashed, I thought of the thousands of small deaths I let myself die in a day—all the many moments in which I am simply not present. Putting on my clothes, sitting at the doctor's office, surfing the web, I let myself miss accumulated days, months, maybe years of my life, as if I were going to live forever. As if being asleep to my life has no consequences.

I once heard a teacher say that returning to our breath is nothing less than reclaiming our lives. I believe he was right. Every time we come back to the breath, we return to our bodies and to this present moment, where our lives are actually taking place.

Practicing mindfulness of the breath is to give sati the reins, as the Buddha said. It is to take it as our ground, our anchor. In fact, I've often used this very image when I'm feeling unfocused, tired, or agitated. On the inhale, I let my hara be suffused with breath. Then I picture the exhale as the anchor holding me steady in the roiling waters of my mind. Resting my awareness on the expansion and contraction of my abdomen, I let all thought, all feeling, all sensation, be held by this breath anchor.

Over the years I've seen there is no storm that my breath cannot weather. Sometimes the waters are calm and my boat steady. Sometimes I find myself in the middle of a hurricane in what feels like a flimsy wooden raft. Yet my experience tells me that I have the ability to ride the waves no matter their size, and that, the closer I get to my breath, the more strength and stability I have.

A Zen poem says:

Rather than give the body relief, give relief to the mind:
When the mind is at peace, the body is not distressed.

The reverse is also true. To give relief to the mind, give relief to the body. When the body is at peace, the mind is not distressed.

In the *Satipatthana Sutta* the Buddha says, "A practitioner trains himself, 'Breathing in, I experience the whole body. Breathing out, I experience the whole body. Breathing in, I calm the bodily formation. Breathing out, I calm the bodily formation.'"

"Experiencing the whole body" can refer to feeling the breath throughout the whole body or to experiencing the breath itself as a body. Inhale, pause, exhale, pause—one body of breath. The instruction to "calm the bodily formation" through the use of breath we all know well. "Breathe," we tell ourselves and each other when we are stressed. The Buddha counsels us to use the breath to calm the body and later on in the sutra, to calm the mind.

During running, mindfulness of breathing will develop your concentration so your mind is quiet and steady. It will increase the fluidity of your movement and help you deal with pain when it arises. And it will encourage you to keep refining right effort so you're not working harder than you need to. Think of the breath as the bridge between body and mind. When your breath is still and even, your body and mind will be steady. When your breath is choppy or laborious, your body and mind will also suffer.

Given this, let's look at the basics of breath so we can use mindfulness of breathing as the fulcrum on which the practice of still running turns.

Abdominal Breathing

Sit upright in a relaxed, comfortable position. Take a moment now to feel your breath. Notice where you feel it most readily: in your abdomen, your chest, your throat? Is your breath short or long, deep or shallow? Does it catch as you inhale, or is it smooth and continuous? Can you pinpoint the moment when either inhale or exhale begins? How about when it ends? Are you aware of the space between the inhalation and exhalation, as well as the space between breaths? Can you feel the rest of your body as you breathe? Do you feel relaxed or tense? Does shifting your posture help you to breathe more easily?

To determine whether you're breathing fully, stand in front of a mirror or ask someone to look at you. Take a few deep, even breaths. Do your shoulders hike up toward your ears? Do your chest or throat feel tight? Do you feel that you can't take a full breath?

Many of us breathe with our chest, using the intercostal muscles that nestle between the ribs, instead of with our abdomen. But these are secondary breathing muscles. They are not designed to carry the load of full respiration. Full breathing is the work of the diaphragm, which acts as a bellows that causes the abdomen to expand on the inhale and contract on the exhale. This motion maximizes the intake of oxygen, which our muscles need to function well.

If you're having difficulty breathing from the abdomen, try the following exercise:

Lie on your back on the floor and bend your knees slightly. Place a pillow under your knees and another under your head. Let your legs relax. Rest one hand flat on your chest, the other on your abdomen just below your rib cage. As you inhale, let your abdomen expand against your hand, and try to keep the hand on your chest as still as possible. On the exhale, let your abdominal muscles contract, again keeping your chest immobile.

Once you get used to breathing this way while lying down, try it sitting and then standing. If you have a desk job, periodically check that you're still breathing with your abdomen. If you feel yourself shrugging your shoulders, consciously relax, and let your abdomen inflate as you inhale. Don't hold your breath—or your stomach. Too many of us breathe poorly out of self-consciousness. We don't want to look fat or flabby. But remember that breath is life energy: if we only half-breathe, we only half-live.

Now let's take the same principles to breathing while running. When you go out for your next run, consciously focus on your abdomen, letting it expand unimpeded on the inhale then contract on the exhale. The most effective way to do this is to focus on the exhale, the active part of respiration, by following the breath all the way to the end, and letting the inhale happen by itself. Then you can introduce a rhythmic breath pattern, as I describe below.

My preferred breath rhythm for running is 2:3 (two steps on the inhale, three on the exhale), but if I'm tired I'll start with 3:4, then switch to 2:3, and finally to 1:2 to sprint. If I need some extra power—while running uphill, for example—I reverse the pattern to 2:1. In general I keep the exhale longer than the inhale so I can empty my lungs before I take the next in-breath, and also because a longer exhale quiets down the stream of thoughts.

Observe the effect that your breath has on your body and mind, but keep your focus relaxed. Controlling your breath will just make you tighter. Remember the lute strings: not too tight that they break, not so loose they won't play. Let your breath be your guide whether you're running, working, or sitting quietly. No matter how familiar you think you are with your breath, there is always more you can learn from it. In fact, you could study the breath for the rest of your life and never exhaust its teachings. It is that vast, that deep, that all-encompassing.

PRACTICE: ABDOMINAL BREATHING

Practice abdominal breathing and establish a consistent breathing pattern while running.

- -

Begin by establishing a running pace that you can maintain with full attention for the duration of your run. In the beginning, this pace may be much slower than you're used to. Later on you'll be able to run faster if you want, but for now you're looking for a rhythm that will allow you to stay relaxed and focused.

Using the hara as the ground or "seat" of your awareness, focus all your attention on your breath as you run. Notice how your abdomen naturally expands as you inhale, then contracts as you exhale. Breathe easily and evenly, placing slightly more attention on the exhale as you let your body inhale by itself.

Unlike Stop-Start Running, in this practice you will continue to run even when you become distracted, which means that building strong concentration will depend on your ability to notice when a thought has taken you away from the breath.

Run at a steady pace, focusing all your attention on your breath. Anchor your mind in it. Let every cell in your body, every thought in your mind, be nothing but breath. When you become distracted, see the thought, set it aside, and come back. Keep running until you feel you are well grounded in the breath.

Now experiment with different breathing patterns to find the one that seems most comfortable for you. Try matching your breath to your steps in a 2:3 or a 3:4 pattern, inhaling for two or three steps and exhaling for three or four. Or try an even 3:3 or 4:4 pattern. Be careful not to hold your breath or let the exhale get too long before you inhale again. If you find yourself gasping for breath, slow down a bit. Walk if you have to. Just stay connected with your breath and your hara. Don't forget your form.

Continue running in this way, maintaining the same rhythm and letting breath permeate more and more of your awareness. Notice when you've drifted away from it out of a habitual need to distract or entertain yourself. Mindfulness of breathing is a very simple, very bare practice. But that is why it is so powerful.

As always, finish with some cooldown stretches, and jot down your observations—when you're first learning these new practices, it's helpful to be able to refer back and see their effect on your running over time.

Not everyone can run, but you can, and you've chosen to. So don't miss the experience as it's actually happening. Allow yourself to be present to your running. Then gradually thread the practice of mindfulness through the whole fabric of your life.

8

Mind

I once asked a group of experienced runners how long they had to
run before they could enter into an effortless, meditative rhythm.

"You mean 'the zone,'" one of them said.

I nodded.

"Four miles," two women said in unison.

Give or take a mile, this is the time needed to work out the
kinks in your body, the restlessness of your mind, the weariness
that makes you wonder why you bother to run day after day when
it is so difficult to get started. But if you're able to get over the
first hump, things begin to flow a bit more smoothly. Your body
grows light and relaxed, and your mind becomes quiet and focused. The space between your thoughts becomes longer; your
movements turn deliberate and graceful. Minutes or miles go by
and you barely notice them. On that rare occasion when circumstances align in just the right way, you may even find you can forget yourself.

The first time this happened to me was on a cold winter evening. I was running on a short country road I often used at night
because of its scant traffic. Just under half a mile long, the road
was straight and sloping, with a single wide curve at the end and a
handful of houses on either side. There were no streetlights, so in
my pocket I carried a small flashlight that I turned on briefly when

the occasional car approached. I didn't want to scare the drivers when they saw me appear out of nowhere.

That particular night there was no moon, so I could barely make out the road. But I enjoyed running like this, more by feel than sight. Going uphill, I focused on lifting my feet and letting my breath go in and out with my steps as I swung my arms easily at my sides. On the way down, I leaned from my ankles and felt my legs turning fast under me. I loved the speed and weightlessness of my body as my feet lightly grazed the bed of dry pine needles lying along the edge of the road.

I kept a steady pace and at first, thought only about random things: a conversation I'd had earlier with a friend, the dinner that was waiting for me, the extra stretches I'd have to do to avoid getting stiff in this weather. Then I began to anticipate the end of my run, particularly the curious thing I knew would happen when I stopped moving. I'd discovered that, when I ran "blind" like this, for a moment or two after stopping my body would feel as if it were still moving. It was a feeling similar to getting off a treadmill. Curious, I'd done some research and found this was due to a kind of vestibular blip. A scrambled message between my brain and inner ear muddled my sense of proprioception— my perception of movement in relationship to the position of my body—fooling my brain into believing I was moving when I was in fact still.

The ear has two otolith organs (from the Greek *oto* for ear and *lith* for stone), the utricle and the saccule, whose job is to monitor the effect of gravity and movement on our bodies. The utricle oversees horizontal movement, while the saccule registers vertical adjustments. Tiny hair cells called mechanoreceptors sit in a gelatinous membrane in both organs. When the head tilts, this membrane is pulled in that direction, causing the hairs to bend. The brain, receiving this information, pairs it with visual cues to determine whether we're standing still, reclining, or moving up, down, forward, or backward.

Most of the time, the communication between my running body and my mind is clear and consistent. I know I'm moving when I'm moving, and my body and mind sense stillness when I stop. But at night the lack of clear visual cues confused my brain into believing that I was the one standing still while the ground "moved" under me, just like on a treadmill. The moment I stopped running, my mind perceived the change as acceleration and told my body that it was now in motion. Then it occurred to me that this kind of sensory mix-up happens all the time, although much more subtly.

As we saw before, the senses perceive the world through sight, hearing, smell, taste, touch, and thought—the six sense consciousnesses. By themselves, the senses *do* have the ability to perceive reality directly. Think of a moment in which you were stunned by a beautiful sunset—the instant before your mind clicked into gear to sort through all its stored images and corresponding labels and put together the concepts "sunset" and "beautiful." Before all that happened—for a fraction of a second, perhaps—you were able to perceive the sunset directly, purely, just as it was. Yet this form of direct perception is rare. Manas, the seventh consciousness, has to process those perceptions in order to make sense of them. It must be able to differentiate a sunset from a fire, a wall from a door, me from you. Further, it can only do so through the lens of the self and its beliefs, assumptions, judgments, and biases. This means that we're constantly sorting, interpreting, and evaluating our experiences, and this cataloging is anything but impartial or objective. It's not direct, and often it's not even accurate.

Then I wondered, how can I ever trust that what I perceive is actually true, especially since most of what is right in front of me I do not see at all? This question led me to remember David, a young blind man who'd come to the monastery to do a monthlong residency.

David, who'd been born blind, had arrived at the monastery with a foldable cane and a mild-mannered black lab—his seeing-eye dog. Despite David's apparent limitations, he adjusted quickly to the routine with minimal help. He always seemed to know where he needed to be and when, and he did any task he was given without complaining—a quality which in itself made him stand out among the residents.

Like many runners, David was tall and thin, light on his feet and full of energy. Unlike most runners, he wore an eye patch. That and his long, dark ponytail often prompted kids to ask him if he was a pirate. After a couple of days of settling in, he approached me and said he'd heard I was a runner.

"Would you run with me?" he asked.

Intrigued, I agreed.

On a mild August afternoon I guided David to the start of the road just outside the monastery's main gate—the same road I had been running on that cold winter night. We interlocked arms at the elbow, and he showed me how I should swing my free arm wide for balance. At first we jogged slowly, but as we got used to each other we gradually increased our pace until we were running at a good clip. By the end of the second week we could race down the road, David's ponytail bouncing on his back and my steps beating time with his.

I wondered what David saw in his mind. I vaguely remember asking him this question, but I can't recall his answer. Yet what I really wanted to know was how he perceived himself in relationship to others and whether, given the choice, he would give up his blindness. I was thinking of a passage I'd read in Annie Dillard's *Pilgrim at Tinker Creek*. She describes how, after a cataract operation that restored the sight of a group of teenagers who'd been blind from birth, a few of them walked around with their eyes closed, yearning for their old blindness. Some of them felt envy, shame, and greed for the first time, and they were so utterly depressed with their newfound sight that they no longer cared whether they lived or died.

Did David consider his blindness a gift or a burden?

Back on my own sightless run, I pulled my neck wrap farther up my face against the growing cold. Lulled by the darkness and the rhythm of my stride and my swinging arms, I gradually let all thought fold into my breath and focused on the *tap tap tap* of my feet on pavement.

Then, in the midst of the stillness and silence, I felt as if a gear clicked into place in my mind, and suddenly I was filled with an overpowering sense of joy and rightness. It was so strong that I actually laughed aloud. The night was right. The road was right, as was my running. *I* was right in a way I had never felt before. In that moment I knew I completely belonged on that road. I belonged to the shadowed pines and the mountain stretching up toward the starless night. I belonged to the biting winter air and the river running full some twenty feet below me. I belonged because I was them and had always been this night, this rhythm, this rightness. How utterly foolish to have ever felt apart, alone, inadequate. How completely impossible.

The feeling faded after a while, but I would encounter it again in my zazen and in the presence of art that awed me.

"I take my waking slow," Theodore Roethke once said. I do too. But I take it willingly.

Right Concentration

Right concentration, or *samyak samadhi*, is the eighth and last factor in the Noble Eightfold Path. The word *samadhi* comes from the Pali prefix *sam*, which means "together" and the root *dha*, "to put or to place." So *samadhi* means "to bring together, to place one's attention single-mindedly on an object." It is concentration to such a degree that subject and object merge. Master Dogen called this the "dropping away of body and mind"—that moment of self-forgetting in which the line between self and other, subject and object, fades. This is why we can speak of "disappearing" into the breath, running, or any other object of our attention.

Samadhi is related to—and in some ways overlaps with— meditative absorption, or *jhana* in Pali. The word *Zen* is derived from this term via the Sanskrit *dhyana* and its Chinese transliteration, *chan.* In the sutras, the Buddha describes right concentration as the attainment of the four jhanas, the ever deeper and increasingly pervading states of concentration that allowed him to gain insight into the nature of the self and reality.

Without concentration, it is difficult to see clearly. It is also difficult to let go of our self-consciousness enough so that we can wholeheartedly immerse ourselves in an activity. That is why Buddhaghosa called right concentration the "profitable unification of mind."

Picture the mind as a lake. When the water is naturally still, we're able to see all the way to the bottom. Every plant, every insect, every stone and pebble, every swimming, skimming, slithering being is clearly visible to our eyes. Likewise, when our minds are still we can see and interpret our thoughts clearly. But if we try to peer into the lake when wind and rain are roiling its surface—when we're caught by strong or disturbing thoughts or emotions—it's unlikely we'll see anything except the disturbance itself.

A single thought is like a rock thrown into that lake. One rock will only slightly disturb the surface, but it won't really affect our overall visibility. A scattering of pebbles will disrupt our view for only a few moments, but if we fling in rock after rock, all we will see is the churning surface of the water and the murky silt obscuring our view.

Because zazen slows down our thinking process, it opens up a space in which we can look at that rock in our hands and decide whether or not to throw it in the water. This means we actually have a choice of where to put our minds. I know this is more easily said than done, but that's why we call it a practice. We repeat, over and over, the process of seeing a thought, letting it go, and coming back to our breath. This is how we strengthen our concentration.

Let me be clear, though, that the point of zazen is not to get rid of thoughts or to stop thinking. The point is to see ourselves clearly. Not every thought is a distraction, nor is there anything inherently wrong with thinking. It's how we respond to these mental formations that determines whether we create further suffering or put an end to it. So an important aspect of practice is being able to discern whether the thought that's just arisen is a thought I need to pick up or a thought I should put down. Is it something I need to let go of, or something I need to acknowledge?

When we carefully study our collection of rocks, we see that they usually follow a pattern. There are the thoughts that take us away from the present moment when we feel bored or uncomfortable. There are thoughts whose purpose is to reestablish our sense of self. Some thoughts are a reenactment of the past, some thoughts project us into the future. We plan, we worry, we anticipate, we distract ourselves, seeking security on ground that is constantly shifting under our feet.

So if concentration is the sharpening factor of meditation, mindfulness is the seeing factor, and equanimity is the balancing factor. Equanimity stabilizes our minds so we can hold difficult thoughts and memories without getting swept up by them.

Acharya Dhammapala, a Sinhalese Buddhist monk and missionary, said, "When there is no equanimity, the offensive actions performed by beings cause oscillation in the mind. And when the mind oscillates, it is impossible to practice the requisites of enlightenment." When we lack equanimity, offensive actions—both others' and our own—create ripples in the mind, like rocks pelting the lake. Without equanimity, it is impossible to practice concentration and mindfulness. Therefore we practice the stilling of those oscillations by riding the waves of our anger, our despair, our excitement and passion. We practice seeing the root of each of these feelings, their arising and passing away. This is how we gradually train ourselves to focus and refine our attention. This is how we become absorbed in our meditation.

In the secular world, this state of absorption is referred to as "flow" or "the zone." Although it's not the same as samadhi, the two concepts are similar enough that it's worth investigating them more closely.

Flow and Samadhi

In the 1990s psychologist Mihaly Csikszentmihalyi described "the zone" as a state of self-forgetting that we experience when performing at peak levels of skill and concentration. He was the first one to describe it as "being in a state of flow."

Flow happens when we become so engrossed in what we're doing, we lose our sense of self. It is the merging of action and awareness.

Athletes who experience flow sometimes describe their concentration as a light beam shining on the activity they're performing while everything else recedes from their field of vision. As their focus increases, their perception of time changes. It seems to either slow down—as in the smooth performance of a particularly difficult task—or to pass so quickly that hours feel like minutes. Finally, in the disappearance of self into action, the action is so effortless it appears to be happening on its own.

In these ways, flow is not unlike samadhi. But the main difference is that flow rarely carries over into other activities; it is dependent on a specialized skill and its matching activity. A master gymnast may be completely focused and able to disappear while executing a challenging routine, yet remain unable to concentrate or cope skillfully in her life at other times. While being in a state of flow is highly enjoyable for the one experiencing it, it doesn't necessarily translate into insight or wisdom. It's only when we couple concentration with insight—"stopping and seeing," as these two aspects of meditation are called in Buddhism—that true clarity and freedom become possible. In Zen, samadhi is single-pointed concentration for the purpose of cultivating insight or wisdom. It is wholehearted immersion in doing for the purpose of seeing clearly the nature of the doer.

There are two main types of samadhi. One is absolute samadhi, the single-pointed attention and self-forgetting that takes place in the perfect stillness of zazen. The other is working samadhi, deep concentration that carries over into activity and therefore functions in everyday life.

Unlike flow, working samadhi operates across activities, regardless of their level of difficulty. We can be fully concentrated while cooking a meal, repairing a car engine, or writing poetry. When we understand that awareness is one continuous thread, we're able to approach any task with full and unselfconscious attention.

Students of the late Bengali teacher Dipa Ma often described her extraordinary ability to be fully immersed in what she was doing, whether she was meditating, teaching, cooking, or hanging the laundry. There seemed to be no break, no bias in her concentration.

Every once in a while, one of these students would complain they didn't have time to practice meditation. "You have time to take a breath, don't you?" Dipa Ma would say in response. "Then breathe with complete attention." She truly believed we could all live our lives aware and awake in every moment. "The only thing that stops you," she'd say, "is your own mind."

In the practice of still running, we train our body and mind in order to clearly see and use that body and mind. Ultimately, we can run to stay healthy or to challenge ourselves. But we can also run to forget ourselves in the simple act of running. In doing so, we can let this self-forgetting teach us something about the nature of who we truly are. This is, by far, the most fulfilling kind of running I know.

PRACTICE: BLIND RUNNING
Run from the inside by running without seeing.

I devised this practice after my runs with David, and I have used it in every running retreat I've led since then. It is the participants' favorite practice—I think because it puts them in touch with a simple but unbridled joy in running.

For this practice you'll need a partner who is roughly your height and runs at a similar speed, as well as a bandana and a path or stretch of road about fifty feet long that is mostly flat and without traffic. A paved road in a park is ideal. You're looking for a smooth surface free of rocks, roots, and any other tripping hazards. Begin with the joint stretches described in the practice called "Your Running Form" on page 58, then run for ten or fifteen minutes until you've warmed up well. Stand on one end of your chosen path or road, and have your partner tie the bandana over your eyes. Make sure you cannot see at all; otherwise the practice won't work.

When you're ready to begin running, interlock arms with your partner. Agree on a signal to start, and together begin jogging slowly so you can get used to each other's pace. As the blind runner, focus on lifting your feet and establishing a smooth stride, and let your partner match your speed. Stop when you reach the end of the road (your partner can let you know when this happens), remove the bandana from your eyes, and jog back to the start. Switch if your partner also wants to try this practice.

Do another blind repetition, this time concentrating on leaning from your ankles and letting your stride open up behind you so you can pick up speed. Swing your free arm wide for balance. Bend your knees slightly, and keep your attention in your hara to stay grounded. Focus strongly on your breath, especially if you feel afraid. Trust your partner.

As you move through each repetition, work on letting go into this trust, and give yourself over to your forward motion. If you're truly running blind, you have no way of knowing where you're stepping or how far you have to go, so allow yourself to stay completely focused on each step as you're taking it.

Depending on how much time you have, move through a few more repetitions so that, by the end, you are both sprinting as fast as you can go. The whole point of this practice is to begin to learn how to disappear into the act of running. It is to run *from the inside*, without thought or measurement. Without holding back.

When you're finished, close with some cooldown stretches. If this practice has worked well, by the end you will feel exhilarated. Remember this feeling—you don't have to run blind to replicate it. Reflect on why you feel this way. So many of us hold ourselves back out of fear of what might be, fear of failing or appearing foolish.

So what would you do, who would you be, if you didn't hold back—if you didn't have a way to compare yourself to others? What would you create or accomplish? Don't be afraid to ask yourself these questions. What you choose to do with the answers is completely up to you. But if you never ask, how will you know?

9

Pain

What is pain? What is its nature? Who is the one who feels the pain, and is the awareness of pain different from the physical sensation?

If you're new to running, let me warn you that at some point, it will hurt. So will zazen. There's really no way to avoid it. As sentient beings we are physiologically wired to feel pain because it is the body's protective mechanism. Pain warns us against possible threats, and if we're injured, it encourages us to remain still so our bodies can heal. But the presence of pain does not always indicate there is something wrong. Even the most flexible or robust person will experience pain or stiffness if she sits or runs long enough. Yet, there is pain and there is pain, and one very important aspect of working with it in the context of spiritual practice is understanding the kind of message that it's sending.

Nociceptors—sensory neurons located throughout the body— respond to three main kinds of threats or "noxious" stimuli: mechanical, thermal, and chemical. If we've broken a bone, been exposed to extreme heat or cold, or ingested poison, nociceptors will send alarm signals to the brain and spinal cord. The resulting painful sensation draws our attention to the injured body part, alerting us to the possible threat so we can protect ourselves.

Depending on the kind of input, pain can manifest as dull aching, sharp stabbing, cramping, stinging, throbbing, irritation, or soreness. It can be acute—temporary but severe—or chronic—milder but ongoing. Paradoxically, our memory for pain is remarkably short-lived. We can vaguely remember images associated with pain we've experienced in the past, but our body mercifully forgets the sensations themselves. This "pain amnesia" allows us to repeatedly, even enthusiastically, place ourselves in situations that we know will cause us pain: getting a tattoo, birthing a child, running a marathon. We know we're going to hurt because we've hurt before, but not remembering the actual feeling of pain prevents us from anticipating and therefore avoiding it.

Yet, in most cases, pain does serve its intended function. A child who sticks a nail in an outlet need only do it once to thoroughly learn her lesson. As uncomfortable as pain can be, there is no question that it is a skillful evolutionary adaptation. In fact, people who suffer from a rare condition called congenital analgesia—the inability to feel pain—are not the better for it: they often suffer from untreated illnesses, broken bones, or infections and tend to have shorter life spans.

Clearly, pain helps us to live longer. But how do we explain those instances when the body experiences pain in the absence of noxious stimuli—on a phantom limb, for example, or while dreaming? No one fully understands the causes of phantom limb pain, but it seems to stem from a kind of neurological tangle. When a limb has been amputated, the brain retains a highly detailed map of the missing limb, creating the sense that it's still present. It then sends signals for the limb to move, but without the matching visual feedback to confirm that this has happened, the brain gets confused. In response, it sounds the body's basic alarm system, giving rise to a painful sensation.

After an injury that led to the amputation of the lower part of his leg and foot, a veteran from the Afghan war said he felt as if his toes were being constantly jabbed with a knife, or like his toenails were being ripped off. In order to help his brain rewire, a physical therapist asked him to sit on an examination table with a mirror next to his good leg. By moving around his intact leg and watching its reflection, the veteran tricked his brain into believing he still had both limbs. In this way he slowly worked his missing leg's overwrought muscles, tendons, and nerves—or at least his brain's conception of them. Over time and with the use of this mirror box therapy, the pain in his phantom limb disappeared.

In recent years, this idea has grown, and biofeedback and virtual reality techniques have been developed to help amputees envision in great detail their missing limbs, therefore reducing their pain. The premise behind these treatments is that, by changing the way the mind sees, the pain can be transformed. This concept is also a key aspect of working with pain during seated or running zazen, so we'll explore it in more detail later in this chapter.

Much more rare than phantom limb pain is pain while dreaming, but those who have experienced it know it can be just as excruciating.

Some years ago I had a dream that I was lying on my bed, awake, though I couldn't see or hear anything. It was as if my head had been tightly wrapped in a thick black cloth. All I could feel was the slow and steady pressure of an invisible hand pushing down on my throat.

Frightened, I tried to move or cry out, but I was completely paralyzed. So I lay helplessly while the pressure on my throat muscles increased and the pain grew from uncomfortable to agonizing to unbearable. Briefly, I wondered if my vocal cords would snap or if I would suffocate first. In the meantime, a remote corner of my brain was struggling frantically to wake itself up, like a swimmer running out of air and kicking madly for the surface. Maybe it was the panic that finally woke me, or maybe the pain triggered something in my brain. The next thing I knew, I was sitting up in bed with my heart pounding and my face and chest drenched in sweat.

Slowly, I got out of bed. I could still feel the lingering shadow of the hand on my throat, but the actual sensation of pressure and the accompanying pain had disappeared. Standing before the bathroom mirror, I looked at my reflection. My throat looked perfectly normal, and if it wasn't for the expression on my face and the memory of the panic I'd felt, I would have thought nothing had happened.

The following morning I went online and found a forum for people suffering from dream pain. I read entries by women and men who were convinced they were being stabbed, crushed, burned, or mangled in their sleep. Some dreamt they were being tattooed against their will or bitten by monkeys. In the worst cases, the pain persisted into waking life. In every instance, the pain's biological cause could not be identified.

It seems that the brain only needs to *believe* that the body is under threat to send pain signals, even if an actual physical stimulus is not present. The good news is that the brain is equally pliable in the other direction. That's why it is possible to work with pain by working with the way our minds perceive it.

But if pain is inevitable for us sentient beings—if there truly is no way to avoid it—is this also the case for suffering?

Pain Is Inevitable, Suffering Is Optional

The Buddha said all human beings experience three main categories of feeling: pleasant, unpleasant, and neutral. It is probably safe to say that most of us would categorize physical pain as an unpleasant feeling. But pain in itself is not the issue. The problem is how we react to it. As the well-known saying goes, "pain is inevitable, suffering is optional."

In a sutra called the *Sallatha Sutta* (The Dart), the Buddha said a person who is upset about physical pain "sorrows, grieves, and laments" over it. This sorrow and lamentation, this resistance and grief, creates a second kind of pain—mental or psychological—which becomes suffering. It is like someone who, pierced by a dart, is immediately hit with a second dart. But rather than trying to understand how this suffering arises, when faced with pain, most of us will either turn away from it or turn toward pleasure to distract ourselves.

Imagine for a moment that you're sitting zazen when your knee begins to hurt. That raw sensation in your kneecap is pain, and by and large, it is inevitable. Suffering, on the other hand, comes with the thought, "I don't like this. I want this pain to go away—right now!" Due to your resistance, your pain is compounded, making the initial pain hurt even more. To deal with this, you try to avoid the pain by adjusting your position. You shift your leg, and the pain subsides—for a while. Then it crops up again, either in the same place or somewhere else. You move again, looking for your sweet spot. You find it, but before long it's no longer sweet. So you move again, fueled by the hope that, if you try hard enough, you'll be able to find a place free of pain. Of course, this place never materializes, so eventually you decide to distract yourself by turning toward pleasure instead. You sit on your cushion, thinking about sex, food, a good movie, and you feel some degree of relief—again, for a while. But sooner or later, the pain recurs.

This endless cycle is inconvenient when we're trying to practice zazen, but it's humbling to realize this is actually how many of us spend our entire lives—moving toward pleasure and away from pain in a constant and futile search for lasting comfort. Yet why shouldn't we believe this is the way to happiness, when it's what our culture promises? Find the right partner, the right house, the right job; work hard to acquire and hold on to the many things you desire; shape your body to conform to society's idea of beauty—*then*, one day, you'll be happy and fulfilled just as you've always dreamed. One day, you'll be able to finally rest. The problem is, not a single person has ever arrived at this imaginary place. Or, if they have reached a state of relative ease, they have not been able to remain there.

Buddhism offers a revolutionary alternative. It says that the sweet spot we're so assiduously looking for is present in this very moment and these exact circumstances. There is nothing we need to change, fix, or avoid. So when pain arises, we don't need to turn away. When pleasure arises, we don't have to cling. This is what zazen is encouraging us to see. It's asking that we allow pain to be pain and pleasure to be pleasure, that we meet each without moving, without resistance or clinging, without fear.

But how do we allow pain to be pain when it *hurts*? What if it's a signal that something *is* wrong? This is where caution and discernment become necessary. If we're sitting zazen, it's important to make sure we're sitting correctly, so it's a good idea to seek the guidance of an instructor. At the same time, we should know that most of the pain we experience is simply discomfort. That is why a central aspect of working with pain is learning to be still within it without turning away from the unease it generates.

There are two main ways to work with pain in zazen, although both are applicable to more general pain management. The first is to move our attention away from the painful sensation. Instead of focusing on it, we focus on the breath. In most cases, this alone will alleviate our discomfort.

Think of a time when you had a bad cold and decided to read a book or watch a movie. Engrossed in a story, you were most likely unaware of your runny nose, your sore throat, your aching head. As long as you didn't focus on your symptoms, they didn't cause you pain. But once the movie ended, once you put down your book, the cold "reappeared." Where did it go when you weren't paying attention to it?

If we want to deliberately practice with pain, instead of distracting ourselves we'll actively redirect our attention. Neither avoiding nor feeding the painful sensation, we will consciously shift our attention to the breath, letting it fill all of our awareness. If we can do this, our experience of the pain will change.

Sometimes the pain is severe enough, however, that we're not able to focus on the breath. Then the approach is to turn toward it instead of away from it. We place all our attention on that raw sensation and *become* it. We get so close to it, focus on it so completely, that we can no longer even call it pain. The gap between the one who's experiencing the painful sensation and the sensation itself disappears.

But let me acknowledge that this way of dealing with pain is counterintuitive. We are so trained to move away from painful feelings or sensations that staying with them requires a great degree of trust and courage.

There's a story about a Buddhist master who was strolling across an open field where a large bull was grazing. At first the animal ignored the man, but as the master got closer the bull raised his big horned head and eyed this two-legged creature with suspicion. The master watched the bull tilt his head as if considering his next move. Then, after a moment or two, the bull snorted a few times, pawed the ground, and got ready to charge. In response, the master lunged at the bull, yelling at the top of his lungs. The beast looked startled for a moment, then spun around and ran off in the opposite direction.

It's not easy to turn toward pain when all we want to do is move away from it. Yet it is our very trust in our ability to work with it differently—the trust that we can face painful, unpleasant, and even frightening experiences—that will prevent us from following the dart of pain with the dart of suffering.

No Pain, No Gain?

When it comes to running, how do we know the difference between pain we can run through and pain we should heed? When is "no pain, no gain" a truism, and when is it an injury waiting to happen?

Every year, between sixty-five and eighty percent of active runners get injured. It's a real concern, and one that many non-runners focus on. "Running is bad for your knees," people often say. I think this is true, but only if we're unaware, overtraining, or running with poor posture. In general, we're not very good at paying attention to our bodies. Even runners can be quite disembodied. That's why slowing down is crucial. We have to be willing to pay close attention to body and mind so we can work with them skillfully.

In addition, there are certain factors that increase every runner's likelihood of getting hurt: doing a lot of hill runs, suddenly increasing mileage, wearing the wrong shoes. Still, I believe it is possible to run safely and consistently. This is what the practical side of still running seeks to address. When it comes to working with pain, we must first learn to identify whether the pain we're experiencing is pain we should heed or pain we can bear. Sudden, sharp, or piercing pain is usually a distress call, while soreness is simply our tired muscles' way of complaining after a good workout. Lactic acid buildup is uncomfortable, but tendonitis can be crippling. A sore knee is manageable; a torn meniscus is not (at least not while running). We can experience raw, dull, or throbbing pain, either constantly or intermittently. Some types of pain are eased with rest; others endure long past the initial injury.

While much of this is obvious, working with pain becomes a subtle practice when the line between healthy and noxious pain is finer. In one sense, some degree of pain *is* needed in order to urge the body past its current limits. The challenge, of course, is to not push your body so far that it breaks like Sona's lute strings. If you're not able to identify the source of your pain, or if it is getting worse over time, err on the side of caution. Stop running and seek medical help. Then rest and let your body heal.

I know how challenging rest can be for many runners. It's hard to remain still when every fiber of our being wants to be moving. But our bodies neither forget nor forgive protracted abuse. In order to create a strong and sustainable running practice, we must base it on clear discernment and right effort. Then, over time, we'll learn when to push, when to relax, when to challenge ourselves, when to be satisfied. Then, having identified and learned how to work with the various kinds of pain that crop up during running, we can turn our attention toward more fundamental questions: What *is* pain? What is its nature?

Jon Kabat-Zinn, creator of the popular Mindfulness-Based Stress Reduction program, encourages those working with chronic pain to ask themselves the following: "Is my awareness of pain in pain?" In other words, is the awareness of pain different from the painful sensation? Or is awareness itself pain? Can shifting our awareness shift our experience? Who is the one feeling the pain?

Yunmen Wenyan was one of the most revered Zen teachers in ninth-century China. The story of his enlightenment experience recounts that when he was still a young monk, he traveled to Muzhou (in present-day Zhejiang) to study with the eccentric Master Muzhou Daoming. After a few days in the monastery, Yunmen went to the master's room to ask for the teachings, but when Muzhou heard Yunmen approaching, he immediately closed the door. Yunmen knocked and stood outside respectfully, his hands palm to palm in gassho.

"Who is it?" said Muzhou through the closed door.

"It's me, Yunmen."

"What do you want?"

"I haven't yet clarified the great matter. I'm coming to ask for the master's instruction," said Yunmen.

Muzhou opened the door a crack, stared at Yunmen, and closed the door again. Yunmen waited for a while, and when it was clear that Muzhou was not going to receive him, he left. Twice he returned, only to be met in the same way. But Yunmen was not so easily deterred. Once more he went to Muzhou's room, and this time he was ready. The moment Muzhou cracked open the door, Yunmen stuck his leg in the doorway.

"Speak! Speak!" yelled Muzhou, grabbing Yunmen by the collar.

Yunmen opened his mouth to answer. Muzhou gave him a shove and said, "Too late!" Then he slammed the door with all his might, breaking Yunmen's leg. In that instant, the young monk experienced enlightenment.

If breaking a bone were all it takes to realize ourselves, we would be living in an enlightened society. So what was different about Yunmen? What did he see? And would he have realized himself if Muzhou had tickled him with a feather?

The koans presented in the Zen literature offer a host of examples of monks attaining realization in ways that seem almost magical. One monk hears the sound of rain, another sees a plum blossom, a third is struck with a stick—or a fist, or a slamming door—and in that instant they become enlightened. Left out of these accounts are the thousands of hours of zazen, the years of spiritual struggle, the piercing doubt these students experienced first. But all of these are implicit in those brief moments of insight. It is only through unstinting discipline, abiding faith, great effort, and even greater determination, that mind and body become ripe for a shift in consciousness, for a new way of seeing self and others. Pain, arising as any other phenomenon arises before the mind, can act as the perfect catalyst for this kind of deep transformation.

Contemporary Buddhist teacher Pema Chödrön has a set of talks titled "When Pain Is the Doorway." The doorway to what? Most of us see pain as an obstacle, but she's saying it's a gate. The only way to experience pain in this way is to turn toward it instead of away from it. The next time you find yourself in pain, be willing to get close to it—so close that you and the pain merge and disappear. If you can do this, you'll get a taste of what the Buddha meant when he said it's possible to put an end to suffering.

PRACTICE: WORKING WITH PAIN
Practice breathing through the pain while running.

- -

Having touched on the ways in which pain can lead us to investigate more deeply its fundamental nature, let me now describe in more detail how to actively work with it when it arises.

If while running you encounter pain, first determine whether it's pain you can work with or pain you need to heed. If it's your run-of-the-mill discomfort—a stitch, a blister, tired legs—the best way to practice with it is by using the breath as your focus. Remember the basic instruction of seated zazen: see a thought, let it go, and return to the breath. Here, the pain takes the place of the thought, so instead of fueling the pain with your attention, you're letting your awareness be filled with breath. Remember that the practice is to neither resist nor ignore the difficulr sensation. Let it be present, but instead of focusing on it, direct your awareness to your breath, gently bringing yourself back to it every time you feel the impulse to move away from your discomfort.

If the pain is strong enough that you cannot redirect your attention, then turn to and breathe *through* the painful sensation. Get close to it, and allow the pain itself to run. Trust that your body and mind can do this. To help you, let your breath be the vehicle with which your body rides the pain. Notice that, the more you can breathe *into* the difficult sensation, the less difficult it will appear. Slow down and shorten your pace if you need to, and again, resist self-defeating or negative thoughts, which will only increase your experience of pain.

If you're struggling with pain during a race, there's another technique you can use to make the pain more manageable. Instead of thinking about the distance you still have to run—the surest way to create suffering for yourself—mentally divide the course into short segments. Choose a landmark about fifty feet away and run to it, still focusing on your breath. When you reach it, choose another landmark and make your way to it. Whether you're in pain or not, don't worry about running a five-, twenty-six-, or fifty-mile race all at once. Focus on covering fifty feet, one step at a time.

In running and in life, being free from pain does not mean escaping from it. It means having the willingness and ability to feel all that we feel—to feel pain without moving away and to feel pleasure without grasping. It means understanding, once and for all, that although pain is inevitable for us human beings, suffering is completely optional.

10

Creation

To heal from illness, win a race, recover from depression, or master a difficult piece of music—these are a few of the many reasons people practice mental imagery. Colloquially known as "visualization," mental imagery actually uses input from all the senses to bring about a desired outcome. An Olympic ski jumper practicing mental imagery will not only "see" the jump in her mind, she will also hear the crowd cheering around her, smell the wet snow, and feel her muscles contracting as she imagines herself performing the perfect jump.

No one would argue that training the body is paramount for any athletic endeavor, but it is now widely understood that training the mind is just as important, because what we think directly affects what we are able to do and what we experience.

Lee Evans, the 1968 Olympic gold medalist who broke the world record for the 400-meter race and held it for twenty years, imagined in detail every single step of that race during the two years leading up to it. Similarly, Billie Jean King, who was ranked Number 1 in women's tennis six times and is, arguably, one of the best female players in history, imagined herself on the court before each game, evoking every detail of the upcoming match. In her mind she'd review her plays in different weather conditions and for various court surfaces (clay, grass, carpet, and hard) and prepare carefully for each one. By the time she arrived at the match, she was as physically and mentally fit as she could possibly be.

Beyond the realm of sports, mental imagery makes it possible to alter our perception in order to create positive change in our lives. A number of psychological studies have shown that people who suffer from social anxiety unwittingly rely on a slew of habitual negative self-images to keep them bound to their fears. Based on assumptions of their social inadequacy, they imagine themselves performing poorly in social situations and then fulfill those expectations when the opportunity to actually interact with others arises. But because this is a learned behavior, it can be unlearned. With the help of a therapist, a socially anxious person can construct a more affirming view of themselves by learning a series of positive mental images. Over time, the new sense of self that these images create changes that person's behavior, which in turn reinforces their self-perception, and so on.

What we think affects how we see ourselves and the world and therefore, what we experience and how we act. Buddhism has known this for millennia, and more recently psychology has been catching up to this fact.

In 1981, in what is now a famous experiment called "Counterclockwise," Harvard social psychologist Ellen Langer took eight men, ages seventy-eight and seventy-nine, to a converted monastery in New Hampshire for a five-day "retreat." The building had been retrofitted to look like a 1959 home, and everything about the space perpetuated the illusion: the paintings on the walls, the shows playing on the black-and-white television, the music on the turntable, even the twenty-year-old photos of the men on the walls (there were no mirrors anywhere). For the duration of the experiment, the eight were to live in 1959 as if it were the present and embody, in every way possible, their younger selves.

The results surprised even Langer and her group of researchers. Before the experiment began, the men had been tested on dexterity, strength, flexibility, hearing, and vision, as well as memory and cognition. When they were tested again five days later, all eight out-performed a same-age control group in posture, dexterity, and even eyesight. In fact, these creaky septuagenarians felt so sprightly at the end of those five days, they started an impromptu touch football game while waiting for the bus that would take them back home.

A Zen expression says, "The three worlds are nothing but mind," which really means that, apart from mind, there is no reality. The three worlds are form, formlessness, and desire, which in essence make up all of existence. That is why Buddhism places such emphasis on mind training. According to this ancient tradition, everything that we experience has its source in the mind.

In the Vajrayana—the tantric school of Buddhism—visualization is called "creation meditation," and its purpose is to realize enlightenment or liberation. At its root is the understanding that we do create reality with our minds, so it behooves us to see things clearly, directly, and as completely as we can. When we don't see, or when we see inaccurately or incompletely, we risk creating suffering for ourselves and others.

The Five Disturbing Emotions

Dzongsar Khyentse Rinpoche, a contemporary Bhutanese teacher, says, "The main purpose of visualization practice is to purify our ordinary, impure perception of the phenomenal world by developing 'pure [or direct] perception.'" This means seeing past the self-serving filters that so often skew our experience.

All of us experience life through a host of emotional filters, many of them negative or "disturbing," as Buddhism calls them. The five main disturbing emotions are greed, pride, aggression, jealousy, and ignorance. Other filters such as dissatisfaction, anxiety, and guilt are variations of these five, but all of them are based on the need to protect our sense of self, and because of this they inevitably create conflict.

Suppose you're running a 10K, and two miles before the end of the race you're leading with another runner close on your heels.

I'll be damned if I let you win, you think as you pick up speed. This is your race. You've worked hard for it, and no one is going to take it from you. This is the arising of greed. With a hundred feet to go, you're still ahead. You see yourself on the podium receiving your medal, signing autographs, being interviewed by the press. Now you are filled with pride. Suddenly, you trip. You stumble and fall, and by the time you get back onto your feet, the other runner has crossed the finish line. Immediately you look for someone to blame. You rail at the universe, the race officials, the runner who is receiving his medal. *My medal, my race,* you think, with your stomach burning. This is aggression coupled with jealousy.

These four filters and their many variations are kept in place by their common denominator, the fifth filter of ignorance. Ignorance is the crank that keeps the wheel of desire and aversion turning. It's the drive that causes us to hold tightly to what we want and avoid what we don't want. Yet, trying to avoid pain and cling to pleasure is not ultimately fulfilling because pain can't be avoided and pleasure doesn't last.

Wallace Stevens said, "It can never be satisfied, the mind, never." In truth, it's the wanting mind, the ignorant mind, that cannot be satisfied. A still, quiet mind does not grasp. A mind that sees clearly is free and at ease. It *can* be satisfied with things as they are. And one aspect of this acceptance is realizing the changing and illusory nature of our emotions.

When we look closely, we see that anger, greed, and jealousy are not solid objects that we can point to or hold. They are like wisps of fog, mutable and ephemeral. This doesn't mean, however, that they're not real. When we feel anger, when our body is flooded with its sensations, when our mind is looping on the accompanying thoughts, and when we take actions to express those thoughts, all of these experiences are all very real to us. But what is the essence of anger?

When we study anger or any other emotion, whether positive or disturbing, we realize that at their core they have no substance.

They arise in an instant and if we let them, they pass away. Neuro-anatomist Jill Bolte Taylor said that the body's chemical processing of an emotion lasts about ninety seconds, but as is true of physical pain and suffering, our reactions to that emotion can enhance and perpetuate it.

From Buddhism's perspective, emotions are, like the rest of phenomena, "empty of self-nature." They are not inherent, they are not fixed, and they certainly do not define us. Working with visualizations helps us to see this more clearly. But visualization is not just positive thinking, and it is not meant to deny, mask, or embellish our anger or pride. Rather, it shows us the nature of an emotion so we can work with it more effectively. In addition, it helps us to cultivate and embody more skillful emotions, such as compassion and equanimity.

For example, a standard visualization practice is to visualize yourself as Kuanyin, the bodhisattva of compassion. First you create a vivid and detailed mental image of Kuanyin. Then, through increased concentration, you become her—you become compassion itself.

In this way, creation meditation works with the limits of the possible, pushing them outward. It channels qualities that are already present in us and deliberately brings them to the fore. The same is true of visualization in sports or any other discipline. If visualization is not positive thinking, even less is it magical thinking. I could spend hours visualizing myself as a world-class runner, but without the training and practice to accompany my intent, my visualization will never move beyond the realm of dreams. The same is true of compassion or wisdom or any other quality we are trying to cultivate.

Further, the images that I use for my visualizations must be meaningful to me. Creating a detailed mental image of the bodhisattva of wisdom, Manjushri, with his killing and life-giving sword would not make sense to a Christian, just as picturing Jesus on the cross would be an ineffective practice for an atheist. An image is never just an image; it is never just a collection of lines and planes. Images create reality because they *are* reality. This means they contain history, meaning, and possibility. The more identified we are with the images we create in our minds, the more transformative those images will be. This is true even when a visualization is unintended.

"Wings of an Eagle"

In 1964 the Sioux runner Billy Mills beat Ron Clarke in the 10,000-meter race at the Tokyo Olympics. It was called one of the greatest upsets in the history of the games, but few people know that it was the direct result of a mental image.

Mills began running when he was seven years old, soon after the death of his mother. He'd read that Olympians were chosen by the gods, so he decided to become an Olympian in order to meet his mother in heaven.

At first Mills was not very fast, but he was determined. He trained and trained, and by the time he reached high school he'd become unbeatable on the track. He won an athletic scholarship to the University of Kansas and was named an All-American three times. But when the student athletes gathered together for a photograph, a reporter asked Mills—the only person of color in the group—to stand aside. This happened, not once, but all three times Mills won the award. The third time, something in him broke.

In his hotel room after the group photo, Mills approached one of the windows, determined to jump. Then he heard a voice inside him that said, "Don't." Four times the voice repeated its plea. To Mills, it was the voice of his father, who'd died when he was twelve. He turned away from the window and wrote down the following wish: "Gold medal. Ten thousand meters." Then he began to train.

Mills qualified for the Olympics, and again he vowed to himself to win the 10,000-meter race. He was virtually unknown at the time, so no one could have predicted that he would actually succeed. Years later, Mills described in an interview what happened during the last eighty-five meters of the race.

With less than a lap to go, Mills was still in third place behind the favorite, Ron Clarke, and Mohammed Gammoudi. But as he was passing a lapped runner, out of the corner of his eye Mills saw the picture of an eagle on the man's jersey. Again Mills heard his father's voice: "If you do these things, son, someday you can have wings of an eagle."

With renewed energy, Mills surged at the last possible moment and overtook Clarke and Gammoudi, winning the race and breaking the world record in the process. He is the only American to have ever won that race to this day.

Afterward, Mills went looking for the lapped runner to thank him, but when he was face-to-face with him, he saw that the man's singlet was blank. "It was simply a perception," Mills said. An illusion whose power changed his life. "And I realized that perceptions create us or destroy us, but we have the opportunity to create our own journey."

Running Visualizations

So how do we use visualizations in our running practice? Because we're working with mind, the possibilities are endless.

Danny Dreyer, author of *Chi Running*, describes visualizing himself as a balloon floating effortlessly up a steep hill during a long run, or "feeling" a bungee cord attached from his abdomen to a target up ahead, pulling him forward. I myself have used water, light, and the deer visualization included in the practice section of this chapter, among others. This last is one of my favorites because it never fails to surprise the runners who try it.

After they warm up and do some light running, I have the participants run up a long, steep hill—the kind that makes you curse with the little breath you have left as you struggle to get to the top.

"Whatever you do, don't stop, and don't walk," I say to them, "even if you think you'd crawl faster. Just keep running."

By the time we're halfway up the hill I can tell they hate me, but because I know what's coming, it's worth it. When we reach the top we turn around and jog down, then I lead them inside and let them settle with a few minutes of zazen. Slowly I guide them through the visualization, encouraging them to imagine and then become a light-footed deer. Then we go back out and run the hill again. Invariably, they are amazed at how much easier, even effortless, the second run is.

All of us create reality with our minds, whether or not we're aware of this fact. Buddhist teachers—starting with the Buddha—have always said that life is like a dream. But it's *our* dream, and there is much we can do to dream it well. Visualizations are one tool to help us take charge of our dreaming. As Billy Mills said, we create and destroy worlds with our minds. Based on our abilities and inclinations—and within certain reasonable limitations—each of us is able to shape our own journey. This is the power of creation meditation.

PRACTICE: DEER VISUALIZATION

Visualize running like a deer.

Before you try this visualization, do a warm-up and then find a long, steep hill. Run all the way to the top without stopping, even if you have to run slowly. When you're done, make your way down and find a quiet space. Read aloud the following visualization, memorizing as many of its details as you're able, for this will make the practice more effective. Alternatively, record it ahead of time and listen to it after your first run. Feel free to add other details if doing so helps you picture the scene in your mind.

Sit comfortably, and close your eyes. Imagine yourself as a deer in a forest clearing. Feel the warm sunshine on your face and the soft grass under you. You've been resting here for some time, and your body and mind feel quiet and relaxed.

Slowly you gather your legs under you and stand on all fours. The tensors in your back legs ripple under your hide as you fully straighten your legs and plant your hooves strongly on the ground. You look around, catching the glimmer of sunlight on leaves and a whiff of something sweet in the air: lavender.

Somewhere out of sight a twig suddenly snaps, and before you have time to think, you are galloping. Your front legs fold and stretch, fold and stretch ahead of you, first the right, then the left, while your powerful hind legs push off the ground together and land ahead of your front legs almost simultaneously. Your torso is perfectly parallel to the ground, its vertical motion imperceptible. With each stride your neck retracts slightly then lengthens, following an even rhythm. You gaze straight ahead as you let your legs turn under you without thought or conscious effort.

You run easily, feeling the wind on the soft down of your face and the joy of speed in your body. Meeting a hill, you lean into the incline and push harder with your hind legs without slowing down. Your hooves dig deeper into the grass as the long muscles in your hindquarters contract and lengthen. Despite your large body, you float uphill as if you were weightless. When you crest the hill your body straightens and you reach slightly with your nose, accelerating even more. It's as if you have been running like this since the beginning of time, every muscle in your body perfectly in tune with motion.

Let this sense of pure movement fill your body for the duration of a few breaths, then slowly open your eyes. Hold the image of the deer in your mind and body as you go out for your second run.

Return to the hill and see if you can bring that sense of lightness into your body as you run it again. See the deer in your mind's eye, and more important, feel yourself become the deer completely.

If you can, do this practice a few more times, allowing yourself to be immersed in the deer's being. When you are finished, let go of the image in your mind before you do some cooldown stretches.

Remember that this power to create reality is always with you. So what will you do with your mind?

11

Stillness

It's summer, and I'm riding the subway in Brooklyn. The car is almost empty, so I can't help but notice the young man sitting across from me. He's about twenty years old, with light brown hair, a square jaw, and worn jeans stretched tightly across muscular thighs. A paperback is propped at an angle on his lap and an old, dirty knapsack slumps at his feet.

At first glance, he looks perfectly ordinary, like an athlete heading off to class or to meet friends at a burger joint. But there's something about him that keeps drawing my attention, and I can't figure out what it is. Then it hits me: outside of a meditation hall, I've never seen anyone sit so still.

Taking a book out of my own bag, I pretend to read while I continue to watch him. His hands, which are resting on his thighs, hold his book lightly. They are perfectly relaxed hands. In fact, every muscle in his body is still and completely free of tension. I glance at the cover of his book. *A Clockwork Orange.* Then I look up and see that his eyes are barely moving. Either he's a slow reader, or he likes to take his time. A few minutes pass before he shifts his right hand just enough to turn the corner of the page, then slowly he returns it to his thigh, and the movement is so slight, it's as if he hasn't moved at all.

It's difficult to describe this level of stillness to someone who hasn't witnessed it firsthand. It's the kind of stillness that pulls you in, like a whirlpool tugging you toward its center. A stillness so complete that right now it seems to envelop me and the whole subway car, the track we're rattling along on, and the busy Brooklyn neighborhood under us, with its jumble of people and cars. It's as if we were all being powerfully drawn into this young man's being.

Several more minutes go by before he again turns a page. I glance at my watch, calculating whether I can afford to go past my stop. I have an absurd desire to watch him get off the train, certain that, given such perfect stillness, his movement will be lithe and graceful and full of power. But I'm already late, so when the car screeches to a halt at the next stop, I reluctantly get up to leave. Slowly I exit the train, then stand on the platform to watch the young man through the window as the train pulls out. Still he doesn't budge. I remain standing until I can't see him anymore, then head toward the exit feeling cheated, like a child who's been pulled out of the theater just before the end of the show. Like I've missed something unique and important.

Further down the platform, a man wearing shades and a bowler hat is playing on a keyboard and singing Stevie Wonder's "Master Blaster." All around him, people hurry by, pressing into the space others have vacated. They move sharply, forcefully, as if afraid of leaving pockets of stillness and silence behind. As if they knew that, without protection, they might just lose themselves—or find themselves—within all of that space and quiet.

Places of Silence and Peace

"In a world of noise, confusion, and conflict, it is necessary for there to be places of silence, inner discipline, and peace: not the peace of mere relaxation but the peace of inner clarity and love based on ascetic renunciation." These are Thomas Merton's words in *Cistercian Life*, a pithy book about monasticism.

Merton understood that in a world increasingly devoted to production and accumulation, to achievement and status, the stark difference and apparent pointlessness of a monastery are its very reason for existing. Philosophers, monks, hermits, and wandering pilgrims have always known that in order to know who we truly are, we must step out of the rushing stream of our lives. We must be willing to stop, reflect, and ask. And we can do this only by resting in spaces where we're able to give up, for a time, our dependence on constant but superficial connection, our insatiable hunger for entertainment and information. To "renounce" here means to be willing to give up our noise and bustle in favor of profound stillness and silence. It means to let go of the endless chatter that covers up our loneliness, and the distraction or overwork that buffers us from our insecurity.

Most of us rush through our days driven by impatience, ambition, or fear. We move faster and faster in our constant effort to do more, acquire more, experience more—even as we buckle under the weight of all the things we need to accomplish in order to "make it." Why be content, our culture demands, when we can be successful? Stress has become our baseline; calm is a luxury to buy at a spa or meditation retreat. Yet throughout history there have always been seekers who've known that our harried way of living is not inevitable. They are those for whom stillness is a right, a necessity, a refuge.

When my brother was in college, I spent a couple of summers with him in Georgia, where he was studying at the Savannah College of Art and Design. He headed off to class early, which meant I had the mornings to myself and could do about an hour of zazen followed by a long run.

On one of those mornings, I was running on a busy street leading away from Forsyth Park when I glimpsed a church connected by an elevated walkway to a plain, squat building on the other side of the street. This second building, whose outer wall was the dirty color of days-old rainwater, had no windows that I could see. But the covered passage joining it to the slightly cheerier church was made entirely of glass, and standing right in the middle of it was a nun dressed in a traditional black habit. Her face was veiled and her arms were folded in front of her stomach, hands hidden inside the long sleeves of her tunic. She stood perfectly still about a foot from the window, facing the world from within her immovability.

My run turned to a jog, then a walk, and about twenty feet from the walkway I stopped and stared. After a moment or two, the nun turned and slowly walked away. She disappeared beyond the edge of the walkway, leaving the glass corridor looking desolate. I waited awhile, but she didn't return. That afternoon, when my brother came home, I told him about her.

"There's always a nun there, day or night," he said. "I've never passed the church without seeing one of them keeping vigil."

Hearing this I was reminded of a story about the Dutch minister and activist Reverend A. J. Muste. During the Vietnam War, Muste stood outside the White House night after night, rain or shine, holding a candle in protest.

One night a reporter asked him, "Reverend, do you really think that by standing here with a candle you're going to change our country's policies?"

Muste replied, "Oh no, sir. You've got it all wrong. I'm not doing this to change the country. I'm doing it so the country won't change me."

Perhaps the nun stood as she did so the world wouldn't change her. Yet I couldn't help but think she also did it in order to change the world. To me, her standing was a clarion call. *Pay attention to all your scurrying*, she seemed to be saying. *You run here and there from morning to night, but do you know why? Do you know where?*

The German mystic Meister Eckhart spoke of the inner and outer work that each of us is called to do, saying that inner work is timeless and sacred. It is the work of silence and stillness, the work of contemplation. Inner work informs and supports our outer work, through which, Eckhart said, our "natural human virtue is expressed." There is no outer work too demanding that well-cultivated inner work cannot help sustain.

One of my favorite anecdotes about His Holiness the Dalai Lama says that once someone asked him how he could possibly have time to do meditation when he is always traveling and has such a busy schedule. The Dalai Lama said, "When I'm very busy, I sit for three hours a day. But when I'm really, really busy, I sit for four hours."

His Holiness understands where his power comes from. He is clear about what he needs to make time for and what is extraneous. But like Merton and Meister Eckhart, he also knows that there is more to inner work than mere quiet and relaxation. The power that comes from deep stillness and that is sustained by single-minded concentration is rooted in the truth of our fundamental nature, in the very fabric of our beings, which is interconnectedness.

Cypress Tree in the Garden

In each of our lives there comes a time when we must choose between sleeping and waking, when we must choose between living or letting life happen to us, between freedom or suffering. And because it is a choice about how to live, we cannot do it just once. It's a choice that we have to make moment by moment, day by day—understanding that what we choose now affects what we choose for tomorrow, and not just my tomorrow or yours, but everyone's. For we are not single islands floating independently in the sea of life. We are more connected, more unified than we realize.

Zen Master Zhaozhou was once asked by a student, "What is the meaning of Bodhidharma's coming from India?" This is a classical Zen question that roughly translates as, "What is the ultimate truth?"

Zhaozhou answered without hesitation, "The cypress tree in the garden."

"Master, please don't teach using objects," the student said. In other words, why are you using things in order to describe the ineffable?

"I'm not teaching using objects," Zhaozhou said calmly.

"Then what is the meaning of Bodhidharma's coming from India?"

Zhaozhou said, "The cypress tree in the garden."

Two hundred years later, a Zen pilgrim is working unremittingly on this koan while he travels through the countryside, visiting various teachers. One night, he stops at a roadside inn and spends the night doing zazen. I picture him in the middle of a deep winter, snow piled high on the inn's inner courtyard and against the building's wood walls. The monk sits alone on the earthen floor of his little room, a woolen robe wrapped tightly around him, his breath visible in the cold air. He sits with complete concentration, with every ounce of awareness focused on Zhaozhou's cypress tree.

Night turns into day, and still the monk doesn't budge from his seat. The air grows colder. Soft footsteps approach the door and after a moment, retreat again. The sun climbs sluggishly up the back of a mountain visible from the monk's room and slowly descends on the opposite side of the sky, but the monk knows none of its movement. Night falls, and the pilgrim continues to sit, his every thought a cypress tree.

Later that night a thief slips in through the monk's window, quiet as a cat, and stands still to let his eyes adjust to the darkness. A passing cloud drifts out of the moon's way, and a beam of yellow light suddenly floods the space. The thief jumps back, startled, for in the middle of the floor, a huge cypress tree stands immovable, its top branches straining against the roof beams.

A moment of total stillness—if it's also a moment of self-forgetting—is a moment in which we recognize that we are irreversibly and inextricably linked to every single being and thing in the universe. And further, that we *are* every single thing and being. We are a grandmother singing a young child to sleep, the steel frame of a high-rise, falling rain on a warm summer night. We are a Wall Street broker, an acre of forest, an oil rig. We are one vast body in which every part is connected to every other part.

From a Buddhist perspective, the "me" that each of us is so invested in—the "me" that we spend so much time and energy building, protecting, and elevating—is nothing but a construct. Underneath it, there's actually nothing that we can point to and call "I." There is simply a collection of elements and an awareness of these elements that creates the illusion of a self that I have learned to identify as "me." Yet, fundamentally, the nature of my self—and of all things—is emptiness, or *shunyata*, "no self." It's not that things don't exist; it's simply that they don't exist independently.

In the *Xinxin Ming*, or "Faith Mind Poem," the seventh-century Zen master Sengcan says, "In this world of suchness / there is neither self nor other-than-self."

"You and I are the same thing," my first teacher used to say. "Yet I'm not you and you're not me." This is one of the fundamental truths that stillness can reveal to us.

Stillness in Zen refers to the absolute realm, the realm of unity, of no separation, of interbeing, where all things are unified as a single whole. Movement is the realm of differences, where you and I are separate and must learn to get along. These two realms work together in perfect harmony in the world of suchness—where everything is just as it is. A monk is a monk, a cypress tree is a cypress tree. But a monk is also a cypress tree, is passing clouds, a gibbous moon. Neither one nor two. Neither self nor other-than-self. If this sounds abstract, we can remind ourselves that all things are constantly embodying this perfect unity between stillness and movement, emptiness and form.

One afternoon I'm running along a deserted gravel road a few miles from home. I keep an easy pace, letting all sorts of sensations drift through my awareness. A warm ray of sun on the back of my neck. The smell of wet grass. The banter between a pair of chickadees just out of sight and the *rat-tat-tat* of a pileated woodpecker hammering a luckless tree for its meal. Under my feet, loose gravel crunches pleasantly with my steps, while all around me the spring peepers are calling out to each other like their lives depend on it.

The path bends and suddenly widens into a clearing. I see a pond in front of me, and at its shallow end a great blue heron is standing, still and stately, on a flat rock half submerged in the water and surrounded by bur reeds. Quietly I crouch where I am, keeping my eyes trained on the bird. She lowers her head toward the water and waits, every fiber of her being intent on the faint shadows flitting just below the water's surface.

She seems almost frozen, except there's nothing fixed about her great animal body. She's gathering herself into herself, waiting for the precise moment to strike, waiting for the exact moment to turn stillness into movement. I crouch in her presence and wait—though not as still, nor as patient. Minutes go by. My legs fall asleep, but I don't want to move. Then, just when I'm about to give up, there's a shift in the air and suddenly the heron is upright, her wings outstretched. With two wingbeats she's airborne, her body rising from the rock where she stood with a movement both light and ponderous. I follow suit and stand up to track her flight until she disappears behind a line of trees at the far end of the pond.

I take a few steps to the edge of the water, pick up a small pebble, and throw it in a gentle arc. It hits the surface with a soft *plop*. I watch the widening ripples expand until their edges collide with the banks and disappear. In the dimming light, I turn and head back home.

Protect Your Mind

When speaking about the importance of inner work, Meister Eckhart said that it requires vigorous commitment to and focus on two things in particular: "The first is that we should have sealed ourselves off internally so that our minds are protected from external images." We must rely on the practice of single-minded concentration. Then, in order to prevent our attention from becoming dissipated or, as he says, "externalized," we should train ourselves to maintain our inwardness. This last instruction is the perfect encapsulation of both zazen and still running. We maintain our inwardness in order to cultivate our own self-power, our own strength. And to do this, we pay special care to protect our minds from distraction.

As we've seen, mindfulness of the breath and visualizations are just two methods of mind training. But there is yet another tool for the cultivation of single-pointed concentration, and that is the use of mantras.

The Sanskrit word *mantra* means "instrument of thought" or "mind protection." It is a sound, syllable, word, or phrase that a practitioner repeats, silently or aloud, during meditation. Called *zhenyan* in Chinese and *shingon* in Japanese, mantras refer to a truth beyond words and meaning, and it's thought that just their sound contains strong spiritual power.

In Buddhism, the repetition of mantras is a common practice. OM MANI PADME HUM—also called the *mani*—is a mantra associated with Avalokiteshvara (another name for Kuanyin, the bodhisattva of compassion). The late Dilgo Khyentse Rinpoche, a highly regarded Tibetan teacher, said the following about mantras in general and the mani in particular: "The recitation of mantra will protect your mind and lead you to realize the wisdom nature of speech. Therefore, recite the mani at all times, until it becomes one with your breathing." He also said that this mantra is the compassionate wisdom of all the buddhas manifested as sound, and that even a single syllable has unimaginable power to liberate and bless all beings.

Simple mantras such as "Buddha, Dharma, Sangha," can be used to still the mind or to develop insight. Ajahn Chah encouraged his monks to recite the word "Buddho" (the Buddha's name) to develop clarity and brightness of mind, saying *bud* on the in-breath and *do* on the out-breath: "The awareness it brings will lead you to understand the truth about your own mind. It's a true refuge, which means that there is both mindfulness and insight present."

Buddhism is not the only religious tradition that makes use of mantras. In certain schools of Hinduism, students undergo an initiation rite in which a teacher offers a secret, personal mantra to guide and ground that student's practice. Some mantras are supplications for health, protection, or a good marriage; some are teachings pointing to the ultimate truth of reality. The mantra *Om* is considered to be the distillation and manifestation of the one reality, Brahma.

The Eastern Orthodox practice of *hesychasm* (Greek for "keeping stillness") incorporates the continuous repetition of the Jesus prayer as a means toward union with God. The prayer—"Lord Jesus Christ, Son of God, have mercy on me"—turns the hesychast's attention inward and keeps the mind focused by containing or limiting both thoughts and input from the senses. Across religious traditions, the senses are often referred to as the "thieves" of our awareness because they rob our attention, causing us to become distracted.

Like mindfulness of breathing, focusing on a mantra concentrates and directs our attention, and this is true in both the religious and secular worlds. Athletes in general, and runners in particular, have used mantras for decades to develop their concentration and generate energy and inspiration.

Joan Benoit, the 1984 winner and record-setter in the first Olympic women's marathon, used the mantra: "The Last Shall Come First, and the First Shall Come Last." During a twenty-four-hour race, ultramarathoner Scott Jurek repeated, "This is what you came for." And the simple but powerful mantra of David Wiley, marathoner and former editor of *Runner's World*, is "Run the mile you're in."

But let me acknowledge again that mantras were originally developed as religious instruments. Their sacred words or sounds are thought to contain great power and to work on various levels, both physical and spiritual. It's only relatively recently that they've been used as psychological slogans. There is nothing wrong with using mantras in this way, but doing so doesn't fully acknowledge their scope, depth, and potentially transformative power. Whether you consider yourself religious or not, be open to the possibility that mantras can be much more than self-help phrases.

In the end, mantras are meant to do exactly what their name says, and what Khyentse Rinpoche described: to protect our minds. "There is nothing more unwieldy or intractable than an untamed mind," the Buddha said. Nothing that leads to such great loss or suffering. On the other hand, through practice and his eventual realization the Buddha discovered that there is nothing that brings more joy or benefit than a tamed mind, nothing that has so much power. So trust the inherent power of your mind, and learn to develop it. Trust and maintain your inwardness, your stillness.

PRACTICE: MOVING INTO STILLNESS

Move into stillness by focusing on a mantra as you run.

To *move into stillness* means to align body and mind, movement and stillness, so they become indistinguishable from one another, like a top spinning in perfect balance.

In this practice we will continue to close the gap between movement and stillness by using a mantra as the point of focus while we run.

Before going out, spend some time jotting down a few phrases you might want to use while running. Then choose one to work with and stay with it for a while so you can get used to the practice of repeating it as you run. If you're not familiar with mantras, I suggest starting with an existing phrase. Later you'll be able to create your own to fit your intent and commitment.

Begin with a short and simple phrase like Wiley's "Run the mile you're in" or "Buddha, Dharma, and Sangha." Part of the practice is figuring out how to match the mantra to your breath and cadence, so begin with a short phrase or even a single word. This will also ensure that you'll remember it, especially when you get tired.

When you're ready to start running, set your timer for five minutes and begin to silently repeat your mantra. If you're using a single word, see whether repeating the mantra continuously—on both the in- and out-breaths—is more effective to keep you focused, or whether it works better to recite on the out-breath only. Either way, let the word or phrase fill all of your awareness. If you notice your mind wandering or if you lose track of what you're saying, stop repeating the mantra for a moment, then start over.

When five minutes are up, relax your mind and keep running for another five minutes in silence. Do this two or more times as the length of your run allows, and notice if your silent running is different after the mantra repetition. I often find that the silence is deeper and more stable after I've been repeating a mantra, and that it becomes increasingly so, until the line between mantra and silence softens and eventually disappears over subsequent rounds of mantra and silence.

If you want to lengthen the time you spend reciting the mantra, shorten your periods of silence. On occasion I will focus on a mantra during an entire run, enjoying the moment when it all falls into place, when breath, body, and words become interfused in my mind.

Don't be discouraged if in the beginning you struggle to keep track of the words or if you find yourself repeating them automatically without much awareness. Gently bring your attention back to your word or phrase, and let both sound and meaning wash over you. Don't try to think about the meaning of the mantra, but be completely attentive to the words. Every time you notice your mind wandering, renew your effort and try again.

As you become more familiar with the repetition of mantras, try using them throughout your day. Notice how different words and sounds affect you and whether their effect varies if you repeat them aloud or silently. Most important, learn about the enormous power that sounds and words have to transform your consciousness.

Gandhi used to say that repeating the name of God has more power in it than an atomic bomb. Given the power that Gandhi himself had, I wouldn't take his words lightly.

12

Movement

Deep in the Nyang-Chu Valley of Central Tibet, in what used to be the kingdom of Ü-Tsang, there's a monastery called Nyangto Kyipuk, the "Happy Cave in the Upper Nyang Valley." Until 1951, when Tibet was incorporated into the People's Republic of China, this monastery was known as one of the two main training centers of the legendary *lüng-gom-pa* runners—monks who were said to "levitate" over the ground as they ran, covering great distances in impossibly short periods of time.

The Tibetan term *lüng* refers to the basic element "air" as well as a being's vital energy (known as *prana* in Sanskrit and *ki* in Japanese). *Gom*, like samadhi, means meditation or single-minded concentration on a specific object to such a degree that subject and object merge. So the lüng-gom-pa are adepts who've learned to harness their breath and vital energy through focused meditation and breathing exercises for the purpose of attaining enlightenment.

The origins of the lüng-gom-pa can be traced to the late thirteenth century, when Tibet's most renowned Buddhist scholar, Buton, supposedly offered his life to Yama, the Lord of Death. In exchange, Buton asked that for the next twelve years all other human beings be exempted from dying. Yama, impressed by Buton's selflessness, decided to spare the scholar's life and instead charged him and his successors with the task of performing a life-furthering ritual. This required that every dozen years a lüng-gom-pa run to all the main shrines and sanctuaries of Ü-Tsang to invite their various protector deities to a special ceremony in honor of Yama. Two centers, the Samding and Nyangto Kyipuk monasteries, were established for the purpose of training and alternately dispatching a runner every twelve years.

There are a number of accounts that describe the lüng-gom-pa's prowess, and they range from the surprising to the fantastical. Yet so few people have actually seen the lüng-gom-pa in action, it is difficult to separate truth from legend. One of the more believable accounts is by John Stevens, author of *The Marathon Monks of Mount Hiei*, who says the lüng-gom-pa could run nonstop for two days, covering over 200 miles a day. An "ordinary" ultramarathon runner set a record of just under 190 miles in twenty-four hours, so it's not outside the possibility that the lüng-gom-pa, given their special training, could run even farther.

Alexandra David-Néel, a French–Belgian explorer and the only Westerner to have witnessed a lüng-gom-pa running, described how they seem to enter a kind of trance as they run these great distances. She recounted that, while crossing the desert, her caravan saw a lüng-gom-pa running in the distance. As he got closer, David-Néel saw the man's ragged maroon robe and the dagger he held in one swinging hand, his other holding up the corner of his robe. His gaze was fixed on a point in the sky far ahead of him, and his steps were so light and regular he seemed to bound over the ground. When David-Néel's servants dismounted their camels to bow to the monk, the man passed them by without a glance, as if he wasn't aware of their presence.

Trying to find out more about these mysterious runners, I read Lama Anagarika Govinda's *The Way of the White Clouds*. In the 1940s Govinda visited Nyangto Kyipuk and described in great detail the history and practices of the lüng-gom-pa. Not surprisingly, their training was extremely rigorous. Candidates could choose to enter a solitary retreat ranging in duration from one month to nine years, and until the completion of their hermitage no one was allowed to see them or interact with them in any way. They lived alone, without name, without family or past, in huts that were sealed from the outside. For food they relied on gifts that visitors offered through a narrow opening in the wall. The lüng-gom-pa could cook the offerings on a small brush-fed fire—their only source of heat during the winter.

The lüng-gom-pa's days were spent studying and practicing breath control exercises and seated and walking meditation. When the training period was over, the seal of the hermitage was broken and the "graduates" emerged to begin their spiritual work as runners, healers, and teachers.

Govinda describes an experience that helped him understand how the lüng-gom-pa could run as they did. During a camping trip with two companions through the lake region bordering Ladakh and Tibet, Govinda went off on his own one day to paint. Several hours went by, and when he finally looked up from his work, he realized that the sun was setting. He was wearing only thin clothes and a pair of sandals, and at first he considered spending the night in one of the neighboring caves. But he'd heard there were wolves roaming about, so he decided he would have to find his way back to camp before it got dark.

Hurriedly, Govinda put away his painting supplies and began picking his way over a boulder-strewn field he'd passed earlier in the day. He jumped from rock to rock for what seemed like miles, struggling to traverse the uneven ground. Not having eaten or drunk anything all day, Govinda was starkly conscious of his thirst and hunger. But uppermost in his mind was his fear. He was certain that, if he stopped to rest even briefly, he wouldn't be able to continue.

After a while, and perhaps by virtue of the repetitive movement of his steps and his heightened awareness, Govinda entered into a kind of trance like the one David-Néel described. All thought and feeling receded to the background until he became conscious only of movement and rhythm. It was as if a strange force had taken over his body, which was moving automatically but with uncanny precision. He was aware but no longer in control. Yet, instead of making him even more fearful, the experience filled Govinda with peace and the certainty that he would make it back to camp safely.

He continued to run like this in the dark, skimming over rocks and picking his way through a swamp without once falling or breaking through the soft ground. Like the lüng-gom-pa, Govinda seemed to be almost floating above the ground as he ran. After a while, he saw the glow of a fire and followed it to his camp, where he collapsed on the ground, utterly exhausted. Concerned, his friends questioned him about what had happened, but Govinda wasn't able to explain how he'd made it back unscathed. He could only describe the feeling he'd had while he ran. His body, suddenly weightless, had moved with a wisdom all its own, and he knew all he had to do was trust it.

I once heard a Zen teacher say, "Just as matter cannot move at the speed of light, the self cannot move at the speed of impermanence."

Einstein's famous mass-energy equivalency equation $E = mc^2$ states that the energy to move a given object is equal to its mass times the speed of light squared. This means that even small amounts of matter require enormous amounts of energy to move. Because energy and mass are equivalent, an object approaching the speed of light will increase in mass, requiring more and more energy to move it. The closer this object approaches the speed of light, the more its energy and mass increase, until they eventually become infinite. That's why an object can never move at the speed of light.

The self is also like this. The more energy we give it, the heavier it becomes, like moving through life with a bag of cement strapped to our backs. The more the lüng-gom-pa forgot themselves, the lighter they became. Perhaps that explains why these monk-runners were able to run the way they did—having shed their weighty sense of self, they were able to move freely at the speed of impermanence.

Gratitude, Not Asceticism

"When you are nothing, then [a sense of oneness with the universe] comes up to fill the space," said a Japanese priest when he was asked why the famous "marathon monks" of Mount Hiei run. Like the lüng-gom-pa training, theirs is a practice of surrendering the self through constant movement.

So-o ("One Who Serves for Others") was the founder of the *kaihogyo*, or marathon monk training, in Japan's Mount Hiei. When he was twenty-five, the young monk had a dream in which a voice told him that the peaks on Mount Hiei were sacred and that he should make a pilgrimage to all the holy places on those mountains, training rigorously like a selfless bodhisattva.

After his dream, So-o built himself a hermitage in the remote Katsuragawa Valley to do a thousand days of austerities. One day, after a particularly intense period of meditation, So-o saw Fudo Myo-o, one of the wrathful protectors of Buddhism, in the midst of a waterfall. Overcome by this vision, So-o leapt into the falls and collided with a large log, which he then dragged out of the water and carved with the image of Fudo. The image was enshrined, and the temple that was built around it became known as Myo-o-in.

As the years went by, So-o acquired a reputation as a wizard and master of the esoteric arts. His prayers, which were often dedicated to Fudo Myo-o, were said to cure terminal illnesses and possessions. After some years, So-o built another temple, Myo-o-do, which became the base for the kaihogyo practice that was developed over several centuries after his death.

The marathon monks—called *gyoja*, or "spiritual athletes"— traditionally began their training by visiting all the holy places of Mount Hiei and doing running circumambulations lasting one hundred, seven hundred, and one thousand days. For their uniform, they wore what became the all-white, mourning garb of the gyoja: a short kimono shirt, pants, hand and leg covers, a long outer robe with a priest's surplice, and a pair of straw sandals. The robe was tied with the "cord of death" into which a knife was tucked, for if a monk failed to complete the prescribed course, he was mandated to kill himself by hanging or self-disembowelment. Then he could use the small coins tucked into his narrow woven hat to pay a boatman to row him across the Sanzu River to the afterlife.

Sennichi Kaihogyo, the thousand-day marathon, remains essentially unchanged from the way it was developed in the 1300s (except the monks are no longer mandated to kill themselves if they fail to complete it). The monk begins his training day at midnight. First is an hour-long service to Fudo Myo-o, his patron bodhisattva. Then, after a light meal of rice balls and miso soup, he starts with a 19- or 25-mile run that takes him through more than two hundred fifty stations of worship throughout the mountain range. Some six and a half hours later, he returns to his starting point for another service to Fudo Myo-o, a bath, and preparation of the noon meal, which consists of little more than noodles, potatoes, tofu, miso soup, and rice or bread. The monk is allowed to rest for an hour and attend to chores, then he must perform another service at three o'clock. Supper is at six, and by eight or nine he is sleeping. This routine is repeated every single day for one hundred days, with the exception of one day in which the run is increased to thirty-three miles on a course that goes through Kyoto.

After one hundred days, the monk can petition to begin the thousand-day challenge, which includes several rounds of one hundred or two hundred consecutive days of running (going up to a distance of 52 miles a day) as well as a seven-and-a-half-day vigil in which he is not allowed to eat, drink, sleep, or rest; a special "home-coming" retreat in which past and present gyoja gather to conduct various ceremonies; and finally, an eight-day vigil in which the gyoja spends every waking hour casting 100,000 prayer sticks into a roaring fire.

Once the gyoja completes the thousand-day challenge, he is considered a Daigyoman Ajari, "Saintly Master of the Highest Practice." As an expression of gratitude, he visits the imperial palace in Kyoto to conduct a special thanksgiving service.

"Gratitude for the teaching of the enlightened ones," said one of the gyoja, "gratitude for the wonders of nature, gratitude for the charity of human beings, gratitude for the opportunity to practice—gratitude, not asceticism, is the principle of the thousand-day kaihogyo."

This is the most important point. The marathon monks and lüng-gom-pa run neither for glory nor penance but for the sake of freedom and self-realization. They move constantly, relentlessly, as an act of praise and devotion, and as a means to realize and express their interdependence with all things.

But short of doing the extreme practices of the gyoja and lüng-gom-pa, how do the rest of us disappear into our running? How do we see that the self is not as solid and binding as we believe it to be? By running with complete attention, with every fiber of our being. By still running, or *just* running. Twenty-five hundred years of Buddhist teachings and history are contained in that word: "just."

In Zen we are encouraged to do each activity with wholehearted attention and presence, without thought of past or future. We just run, just sit, just work, just eat, just rest. And although it seems like it should be easy to just do what we're doing, as we're doing it, it's actually extremely difficult—almost impossible without some kind of practice—because our minds are so insistently and enthusiastically distracted.

I myself have spent decades training myself to just run—to run as simply and unselfconsciously as possible—a fact I find both ironic and fitting. As Moravec said, often it is the simplest tasks that require the most practice to do effortlessly—unless, like ultramarathoner Diane Van Deren, you receive some unexpected help from fate.

When Diane Van Deren was in her twenties, she was diagnosed with epilepsy. But as a longtime runner, she discovered that if she went out for a run just as she began to feel a seizure coming on, she could prevent it. For years, every time Van Deren felt the onset of a seizure she'd run out the door, telling her children that if she wasn't back in five hours they should call an ambulance.

But the seizures increased in strength and frequency, and after a while Van Deren was no longer able to outrun them. After consulting her doctors, she decided to have a lobectomy that removed a section of her brain and effectively halted the seizures. Yet, in their place appeared a series of side effects that Van Deren had to learn to adjust to.

Van Deren cannot read a map, has trouble getting organized and remembering even simple facts, and has largely lost her sense of time. And while these side effects make Van Deren's daily life challenging, they also turned her into an unparalleled long-distance runner.

Since her operation, Van Deren can quite literally run on and on. She can't track her pace or her mileage, which means she never worries about how long she's run or how far she still has to go. She simply runs, listening to the sound of her breath and the natural rhythm of her footsteps.

I'm certain that Van Deren's life is not easy, but at least in her running she is utterly free. She truly just runs. For the rest of us, I wonder whether our increasing inability to focus—our inability to find rest *within* the activity of our lives—is the main reason we are often so stressed, so exhausted.

Yet it's never too late to retrain ourselves to stay focused and alert; to do what we're doing wholeheartedly. When we give ourselves completely to what is directly in front of us—whether that's a run, a work project, a difficult conversation—and gradually let go of the self, we begin to realize that no one's put that bag of cement on our backs. We picked it up, and year after year we carry it around, adding more weight as we let our beliefs, opinions, and worries become increasingly solidified. As the Buddha saw, it doesn't have to be this way. All of us can learn to see that the self is not as solid or as heavy as we think. When we realize that it is simply a construct, an idea we maintain with an inordinate amount of energy and time, then we can choose to set it down. We can choose to live lightly, with joy and ease.

PRACTICE: STILL RUNNING
Practice still running at least once a week.

This practice picks up where the previous one left off and takes it a step further. Now, instead of using a mantra to keep you anchored within your running, you'll let go of even that subtle aid and *just* run. All of the tools, all of the posture guidelines and breath exercises and concentration practices, are firmly under your belt. It's time to let them go and give yourself over to still running.

Like the practice of blind running, still running demands a great degree of trust. Trust that our bodies know what to do. Trust that our minds can quiet down and remain focused and aware. Trust that whatever level of energy we think we have will be enough. And that, even if we don't have energy, *that* is enough too.

After moving through the joint stretches in the practice called "Your Running Form" on page 58, set your timer for thirty minutes or so and begin running slowly. If you're running indoors, don't turn on the TV. Don't talk on your cell phone, surf the web, or listen to music (this last goes for running outdoors as well). Don't read a book or flip through a magazine. Allow all of your attention, all of your energy, to go into the simple act of running.

Without focusing on anything in particular, keep your awareness clear and open. Notice any thoughts or images that move through your mind. Be aware of sensations in your body, as well as your environment. If you're tired, slow down, but keep your attention clear. If you notice yourself speeding up in order to finish your run, again slow down enough to pay attention to what you're doing. Don't go on autopilot.

Notice your breath, but don't force it into a pattern. Just observe what it's doing without trying to manage it in any way. Notice what happens as you shift your gaze, especially if you're running outside. The lüng-gom-pa look up, fixing their attention on a distant point in the sky. The marathon monks gaze straight ahead at a point about a hundred feet in front of them. What happens when you do either one? What happens when you look just a few feet ahead of you?

If you need to adjust your form, do so, but don't keep tinkering with it. At this point you want to let go of the mechanics of running and experience it as the art that it is. There is no particular way that this practice should feel. Rest in the open awareness of your mind, in the fluid movement of your body. Do not try to do anything, get anywhere. After moving into stillness, we're now letting that stillness permeate our movement in such a way that the two become indistinguishable. This is where running and zazen truly merge.

Continue still running until the end of the time you set for yourself, then take ten or fifteen minutes to stretch and cool down.

If you find yourself tuning out during this practice, start with a shorter run next time. If you need to, focus on your form or your breath and leave the last ten minutes to just run. It's better to run with complete attention for ten minutes than to run mindlessly for an hour. Slowly build on the concentration you've been cultivating, keeping yourself challenged and engaged for the duration of a run. Little by little, you'll feel your body relaxing, your mind quieting down, your attention sharpening. Just as with zazen, after a while you won't need to work so hard to stay present.

After attending my running workshops some runners ask whether it's bad form to run with music. No, it isn't. I myself prefer to run without distractions, to really practice running zazen, but if after trying these practices you decide that you miss listening to music while you run, that's fine. What you do is completely up to you. Just choose deliberately. Choose to be awake in all the many and varied moments of your life so that, in the end, hopefully you'll be able to look back at that life and say, *It wasn't perfect, but I was there for it.*

13

Silence

We live in a world of constant communication. Yet it doesn't seem to matter anymore whether that communication is skillful or divisive, true or false. Words are cheaper than ever, and like consumers chasing after a good bargain, we can buy them wholesale without looking too closely at what it is we're getting. But we can also choose to be more selective, more careful about what we offer and what we take in. We can be ever more aware of how our words affect us and others, how they help to shape the reality that we're living in.

Silence is not just the opposite of speech; silence also creates a space to discern what is needed when relating to others. It helps us to pause and ask ourselves whether the most appropriate choice is to speak up or keep quiet. If we choose to speak, silence gives us the opportunity to weigh our words carefully.

I often think of the practice of silence in terms of the first of Buddhism's Three Pure Precepts, the moral and ethical principles that guide an awakened life: refraining from harm, practicing good, and actualizing good for others. From the perspective of the Three Pure Precepts, choosing silence means to not create harm with our words. It means to refrain from speech that is divisive, unskillful, false, or idle. To practice good means to practice *right speech*—one of the factors in the Noble Eightfold Path—by offering words that are kind, skillful, and appropriate. And to actualize good for others means to carefully choose words whose purpose is to help rather than harm, to elevate rather than denigrate. Even when we're not able to be more proactive, at the very least we can give up our desire to hurt others with our words. We can renounce our right to lash out when we feel attacked or insulted. Choosing silence in such moments means suspending our belief that our identity or pride is paramount, and that showing others where they've gone wrong is our responsibility. That's why, if we're going to walk a spiritual path, our desire to be clear must be stronger than our desire to be right.

There's a Zen story about a teacher who was known for the severity of his ascetic practice. He spent all his time alone in a mountain hermitage, but as inevitably happens with people like him, word got out about his spiritual power, and an intrepid student tracked the master to his little hut. For days the hermit ignored the young woman, who hung around him and watched him intently as he went about his tasks. To her disappointment, the old man seemed perfectly ordinary. He showed no signs of the kind of discipline she had expected of him. He got up—rather late, she thought—washed his face, ate a small meal, cut some firewood, walked quietly, meditated for a little while, ate some more, rested, read and wrote, sat quietly again. Where in the world had all those stories about his uncompromising rigor come from?

A few more days went by, and the student tried unsuccessfully to engage the master in conversation. Finally, as the old man was going out to fetch water one morning, she blocked his path. Surprised, he looked at her as if she were a tree that had uprooted itself to stand before him. But it was not an unkind look, so she felt encouraged and quickly blurted out, "Please, I just want to ask you one question. I've heard of your strong ascetic practice, but all I see is a hermit eating food and drinking water. Tell me, what *is* your ascetic practice?"

"My ascetic practice?" the hermit repeated thoughtfully. "My ascetic practice is that I don't deceive myself."

The practice of silence demands that we stay true to ourselves and to circumstances. It asks that we see clearly and that we speak or refrain based on what we see. But the dark side of silence is that we can hide within it or use it to oppress or collude. So to practice "noble silence," as the Buddha called it, requires a great degree of honesty. It requires that we know when to speak and why.

In a passage in the *Kolita Sutta*, Maudgalyayana, one of the Buddha's foremost disciples, wonders aloud what the nature of noble silence is. "I hear the phrase all the time," he says to himself. "'Noble silence,' 'noble silence'—but what *is* noble silence?" And then he himself answers, "There is the case where a practitioner, with the stilling of directed thought and evaluation, enters and remains in the second *jhana*: rapture and pleasure born of concentration, unification of awareness free from directed thought and evaluation—internal assurance. This is called 'noble silence.'"

After spending some time in meditation, Maudgalyayana comes to the conclusion that noble silence is tantamount to the unified awareness and "internal assurance" that a practitioner attains in the second jhana. (There are four main jhanas, or progressively deeper states of concentration, in which subject and object, process and goal, effort and relaxation, become ever more subsumed into one another until all distinctions between them disappear.) In the first jhana, a practitioner deliberately directs her thoughts and continually brings herself back to the object of her meditation. It's a practice that requires great effort and single-minded attention. In the second jhana this process happens effortlessly, just as a lake without outflow gradually fills when water pours into it. Without directed thought, without any kind of evaluation, the mind settles naturally into unified awareness, leading to clarity and insight. This, Maudgalyayana says, is noble silence.

Much of zazen is learning to become familiar and comfortable with deep silence. As with stillness, silence is cultivated, not for the sake of silence itself, but to create space for our natural, clear, bright mind to reveal itself. Although this mind is always present, it is often clouded by our thoughts and strong emotions, by our worry and anticipation. But there is a way to rest in this mind. And this, we could say, is the natural way of sustaining our meditation.

Six Ways of Resting

Sometime in the tenth century, an Indian Buddhist master by the name of Tilopa gave a teaching called the "six points for sustaining meditation" or "six ways of resting": do not recall, do not think, do not anticipate, do not meditate, do not analyze, *do* rest naturally.

"Do not recall" refers to not getting tangled up with the past during the time of meditation. The past no longer exists. It is like a corpse, without life or will, so there is no point in recalling it. The future hasn't been born yet, so it is equally pointless to dwell on it. Therefore, *do not anticipate*. Even the present becomes the past once we've lived the moment. So don't get lost in ideas of time, Tilopa says. Don't worry about what was or what will be. And *do not think* about what is happening now because it won't help you to be more awake.

A century before Tilopa's time, a young Chinese monk named Deshan Xuanjian decided to travel south in order to spread the teachings of the *Diamond Sutra*. Having heard that Zen practitioners in the south "do not rely on words and letters," he wanted to set them straight. So he wrapped up all his sutra commentaries in a bundle and set out walking. After several weeks of traveling and teaching, Deshan came upon a small roadside stall where an old woman was selling cakes and tea. Hungry and weary, Deshan asked her for some refreshments.

"Sure," said the old woman, "but before I serve you, Reverend, can you tell me what you are carrying on your back?"

Deshan stood a little straighter and said, "These are important commentaries on the *Diamond Sutra*. There is no part of this text that I myself have not mastered. You may have heard of me. They call me 'Diamond Zhou.'"

"Oh, this is so fortuitous," the old woman said. "May I ask you a question?"

"Of course," Deshan set down his bundle and took a seat in front of the tea seller, ready to hold forth.

"I've heard that in this sutra it says, 'Past mind cannot be grasped, present mind cannot be grasped, future mind cannot be grasped.' Is that so, Reverend?"

"Yes, that is correct," Deshan said indulgently.

"Then tell me, with which mind will you eat this cake?"

Deshan was speechless.

In one version of the story, the monk then asked the old woman to direct him to a Zen master—completely missing the one standing in front of him. The old woman humbly sent him to a nearby monastery, where after a long conversation with the teacher, Deshan had an awakening. In another version, the tea seller flipped her sleeves in contempt and left Deshan where he was, tea-less and cake-less.

But her question remains. With which mind will Deshan eat his cake? With which mind are you reading this book? The answer to this question can only be accessed through noble silence, through the unification of awareness free from directed thought and evaluation. Only through still and silent contemplation can we gain internal assurance—a quiet, nonintellectual kind of knowledge.

Next, Tilopa says, *do not meditate*. But isn't that the whole point of meditation—to meditate? Not when doing so complicates the simple act of resting in awareness, resting on the breath. Master Dogen said, "The zazen I speak of is not learning meditation. It is simply the dharma gate of repose and bliss, the practice-realization of totally culminated enlightenment. It is the manifestation of ultimate reality." Zazen is the manifestation of reality. Therefore, to not meditate means to trust each moment as it is, without any need for intervention. This is one of the most difficult points to accept about meditation: we practice long and hard in order to learn how to let go of practice. We exert effort in order to achieve effortlessness.

Do not analyze means to not judge your state of mind or the quality of your meditation. Don't get frustrated when your mind won't settle. Don't get excited or restless or fearful when you start to get quiet. Don't criticize, don't measure, don't compare this meditation period to another. Don't wonder when you'll achieve enlightenment or how it will feel when you get there. Don't let even the slightest movement, the slightest thought separate you from that natural, clear, bright mind.

Many years ago I was working on a koan with my teacher. I had been struggling to see it for quite a while, and every time I went into the *dokusan* room to present my understanding, my teacher unceremoniously rejected my answers. Month after month I sat with the question in my zazen, striving to see what the koan was pointing to. But every time I went before my teacher he just shook his head and rang the bell that terminates the interview. Finally, at my wit's end, I cried out at the end of one of these meetings, "But why am I having such trouble with this?!" My teacher smiled and calmly said, just before ringing his bell again, "Because Vanessa *needs to know.*"

He was right, of course. I didn't know how to *not* know, how to not measure my progress or look for answers. It was years before I would learn to truly rest in body and mind.

Do rest naturally means resting with and in mind just as it is. Without creating, without fixing, mind rests in mind's own nature, which is bright, luminous, and free. With or without practice, with or without effort, mind is always clear and bright. But practice and effort are required in order to see this. We must cultivate deep stillness and silence because we can't rest in mind when we're talking to ourselves, while we're busy worrying, planning, judging, or remembering.

So think of silence as the still, open space of that bright mind, while noise is its clutter. Whether inner or outer, noisy places are chaotic. They make us feel ungrounded and cut off from one another. It's not an accident that all spiritual traditions with strong contemplative practices have a solid grounding on the practice of silence.

But what is silence itself? The moment we speak of it, we break it. When we try to define it, we move away from it. Silence, like light, is usually understood by virtue of what surrounds it. Just as we can see light only by observing the objects it illuminates, we identify silence by contrasting it with sound or noise. There is, objectively, no such thing as perfect, absolute silence in our world. And yet, silence can clearly be felt, which means it is not just the absence of sound. Silence is palpable and full of presence. We all recognize it, some of us crave it, many of us fear it. But I think Pascal was right when he said that all of humanity's problems stem from our inability to sit quietly with ourselves. For it is through the silence and stillness of contemplation that we learn to be *in* and *with* the world. We learn to be with ourselves so we can be with others. We learn to see and be seen.

Seen by Another

Not long after arriving at the monastery I was running on a country road on a hot summer day. The midday sun beat down on my face and arms, and I both welcomed and resisted it. My body usually loves running in the heat. My mind, on the other hand, loves to complain, and this particular day it was in fine form. *It's too hot. You shouldn't be running. You're already tired. And thirsty. This is stupid. Why don't you just go home?*

I moved slowly, feeling the sweat pool on my hairline and slowly drip down my nose. I tried telling my body it wasn't that hot or tired, but it had passed its threshold and would no longer listen. Finally, I gave up thinking and just focused on the sound of my feet on asphalt. On either side of me, the acres of farmland crawled past.

Having stopped talking to myself, I then became aware of the quiet around me. I couldn't hear a single sound—not a car, tractor, or chainsaw. There were no birds chirping or insects trilling, and no breeze either. I was running in a silence so thick I could almost touch it.

Slowing down even more, I looked around, searching for any signs of life. A dog running across a yard or chickens pecking at the ground. Kids playing. Voices behind an open window as I passed by. There was nothing.

Where in the world is everyone? I thought.

Suddenly I was seized with the strangest feeling. I felt as if I was a character in a Haruki Murakami novel. As if I'd walked through an invisible portal and entered a parallel universe where I was the only living being left on earth. Or maybe I'd died and hadn't yet realized it.

I knew I was being foolish, but I felt a flicker of fear nonetheless. I quickened my pace and tried to focus on my breath. Surely if I was still breathing that meant I hadn't died. I passed a young maple and out of the corner of my eye, saw movement. On a low branch was a Carolina wren, flicking his wings as if he were cleaning them. When I got close he stopped and looked at me knowingly. I returned his look, grateful for the acknowledgment. I existed because I had been seen—or so it seemed to me in that moment.

Right, left, right, left. I continued to place one foot in front of the other as I ran, the wren now behind me. Above me, bands of cirrus clouds streaked the sky like marks from a painter's brush. To my left, a newly painted yellow barn stood slightly away from the road, on its peak a dark weathercock standing perfectly still, its beak open as if singing a song only it could hear.

PRACTICE: JUST SITTING

Just sit in silent, open awareness.

- -

This is the last practice in the book, and it is not one that involves running. The reason is that I want to leave you in the power and spaciousness of just sitting. As in the previous practice, you are no longer trying to *do* anything when you practice this form of zazen. Do not strive to focus your mind, direct your thoughts, or even gain insight. The practice here is to simply sit silently and openly with what is.

If you can set aside at least half an hour a day for this practice, that's ideal, but even ten minutes of silent sitting each morning or evening will have an effect on your body and mind.

Settle into your usual zazen posture, and this time close your eyes. Hold your hands in the zazen mudra, or rest them on your knees or lap. Take a few breaths, concentrating on the rise and fall of your abdomen. Once you feel grounded, move your attention to your ears. Listen closely. See if you can listen *into* the silence itself, letting your mind rest within it. If you feel the impulse to label the sounds you're hearing, relax your awareness and return to just listening.

Now let your attention become more open so you can take in other impressions: thoughts, feelings, smells. Allow them to arise in your mind, watch them persist for a moment, then let them pass away. Sit in their presence without trying to change or manipulate them.

Remember that there isn't a single thing that is not you, that is not mind. This means you don't have to turn away, you don't have to fix or reject any thought, any feeling, any sensation. Simply be with what is. Allow your zazen to be spacious and free. To help you, use Tilopa's six ways of resting: do not recall, do not think, do not anticipate, do not meditate, do not analyze, *do* rest naturally in the clear, bright, natural mind.

When the time is up, stand up slowly, taking care not to disturb your quiet so you can carry it into the rest of your day.

I believe it is more important than ever that we protect silence as a vital yet increasingly rare resource. Because it is only in silent places that we'll be able to cultivate the peace of inner clarity and love.

14

Credo

As I come to the end of this book, let me return to the premise I began with: it is possible to live an awake and fulfilling life, and as human beings, we have everything we need to do so.

We have the power of stillness and silence and the dynamism of clear, unhindered movement. We have healthy bodies—healthy enough at least to consider running as a practice—and we have human consciousness. All we need is to cultivate our desire to wake up. Our desire to be free.

The truth is, the world doesn't need faster runners. But it desperately needs people who are clear and awake. Zazen, whether moving or still, can help us cultivate that clarity and wakefulness.

I often think of zazen as the candle that Reverend Muste held, night after night, outside the White House. When I sit in stillness and silence, I am declaring my intent to not let myself be changed by the world, not to be shaped in its image. Quietly, I turn inward in order to determine the kind of life I want to live instead of playing out a pattern dictated by others. When I practice moving zazen I resist being swept up by the current of grasping and gaining and fighting and accumulating that drives so much of our actions as human beings—actions that Buddhism recognizes are fueled by ignorance. Ultimately, I believe that same ignorance will never be commensurate with our ability to learn, reflect, and act according to what is true and life-giving.

I believe that zazen is more powerful than the sum of our human intelligence, our physical strength, and our will. It is more powerful because it reveals the truth of who we are in relationship to every other created thing. It shows that fundamentally we are indivisible.

I believe in our awakened nature and in our capacity for wisdom and kindness. I believe that, when we don't act out of these qualities, it's not because we're lacking in any way, but because we suffer from a kind of temporary amnesia. In our rushing about, in our looking outward for validation, we forget that clarity and love, joy and balance, are the very fabric of our being, our ground and inheritance.

I believe that what we think is what we do, and what we do is who we are. I believe that stillness and silence create the space we need to understand these truths.

I believe in our courage, our resilience, our insatiable curiosity.

I believe that, until the last day that humans walk on this earth, there will always be seekers who will not go halfway, who will not be satisfied with easy answers. These seekers understand that there is no such thing as the pursuit of happiness, because each and every moment is an arrival. And more, that happiness is not true happiness until it is everyone's.

That is why, in the end, I believe we would rather be clear than be right. I believe that in our search for peace and freedom, for basic love and dignity, we will always be unstoppable.

This I believe with all my heart.

Acknowledgments

All my gratitude to my teachers, John Daido Loori Roshi and Geoffrey Shugen Arnold Roshi, and to my parents, Eduardo and Cristina Goddard. For your many teachings, your love, and most important, the gift of life—thank you.

Gratitude to Shideh Tenkei Lennon, Chris Tyler, Luca Mokudo Valentino, Danica Shoan Ankele, Shea Zuiko Settimi, Valerie Meiju Linet, Steven Seigan Miron, and Ben Ehrlich. Carefully reading and commenting on a developing manuscript is the least of it. Each of you offered me what any writer dreams of: kind yet unstinting advice and encouragement. Gratitude also to Dora King for your keen eye and your deep and loving stillness and silence.

Gratitude to Rachel Neumann and Audra Figgins, without whom this book would not have made it past an idea, and to the staff at Shambhala Publications for their dedication to making the dharma teachings widely available.

Finally, to quote again the wise words of a marathon monk: "Gratitude for the teaching of the enlightened ones, gratitude for the wonders of nature, gratitude for the charity of human beings, gratitude for the opportunity to practice."

Glossary

C. Chinese
G. Greek
J. Japanese
P. Pali
S. Sanskrit
T. Tibetan

abdominal breathing Also called "diaphragmatic breathing"; the natural and relaxed form of breathing of all mammals. It occurs when the diaphragm, as opposed to the secondary chest muscles, contracts in respiration.

absolute In Buddhism, one of the aspects of reality; refers to oneness or emptiness (*shunyata*). It is dependent on and mutually arising with the relative, the physical manifestation of emptiness.

absolute *samadhi* Single-pointedness of mind achieved during deep states of concentration in seated meditation; stands in contrast to relative *samadhi*, which occurs during activity, e.g., during walking meditation.

alaya-vijñana (S.) The storehouse consciousness; the eighth of the eight types of consciousness in the Yogachara school. It contains all the seeds of our actions that will potentially "bloom" into particular effects.

anapanasati (P.) "Mindfulness of inhalation and exhalation" or "mindfulness of breathing." A foundational Buddhist method of meditation that requires sustained focus on the act of breathing.

awakening *See* enlightenment.

Bodhidharma A fifth- or sixth-century monk credited with taking Buddhism from India to China and founding the practice of Shaolin kung fu. The phrase "What is the meaning of Bodhidharma's (or the Ancestor's) coming from the West?" essentially means, "What is the meaning of Zen?" or "What is the ultimate truth?"

bodhisattva (S.) Literally, "enlightenment being." One who has vowed to postpone their own enlightenment for the sake of helping others to attain the same. In Buddhism there are a number of bodhisattvas, such as Avalokiteshvara or Kuanyin, the bodhisattva of compassion; Manjushri, the bodhisattva of wisdom; and Samantabhadra, the bodhisattva of wisdom in action.

Buddha (c. 563–483 BCE or c. 480–400 BCE). Siddhartha Gautama. After six years of rigorous practice he attained enlightenment under the Bodhi Tree and then taught the tenets of Buddhism for the next half-century. Also a person who is enlightened.

Buddhaghosa A fifth-century Indian Buddhist commentator, translator, and philosopher. Best known for the *Visuddhimagga,* or *Path of Purification.*

Buton (1290–1364) Buton Rinchen Drob, Tibet's most renowned historian and scholar, as well as the abbot of Shalu Monastery.

Chan (C.) *See* Zen.

concentration *See* samadhi.

dantian (C.) *See* hara.

Deshan Xuanjian (780–865 CE) A ninth-century Chinese Zen master known for his fierceness. In his early years he had a reputation as an expert in the *Diamond Sutra,* a Mahayana text.

dharma (S.) "Factor," "element," or "phenomena"; also "truth," "doctrine," and more specifically, the Buddha's teaching.

dhyana (S.) *See* zazen.

diaphragmatic breathing *See* abdominal breathing.

emptiness The absolute basis of reality; lack of intrinsic nature or independent existence.

enlightenment Seeing into the nature of the self and of reality; realization; "seeing things as they are." Also *nirvana*, or "cessation" from the endless cycle of existence that leads to suffering.

"Faith Mind Poem" *Xinxin Ming.* Poem written by sixth-century Chinese Zen master Sengcan, famous for its opening sentence: "The Great Way is not difficult, just avoid picking and choosing."

flow A term coined in the 1970s by psychologist Mihaly Csikszentmihalyi. It denotes a state of mind in which a person is fully focused on an activity to the exclusion of everything else.

Fudo Myo-o One of the Five Wisdom Kings in Buddhism; his fierceness is said to dispel away the defilements that prevent a seeker from reaching enlightenment.

gassho (J.) A hand position—palms together and fingers pointing upward in front of the chest—that in Buddhism expresses gratitude and reverence. It is also a greeting and a sign of humility.

hara (J.) "Abdomen." In Japanese medicine and martial arts, the *hara* is both an anatomical area and a powerful field of energy used in the practice of concentration.

hesychasm (G.) From the Greek *hesychia*, meaning "stillness, rest, silence." A contemplative form of meditation in the Eastern Orthodox Church, consisting of repeating the Jesus Prayer ("Lord Jesus Christ, Son of God, have mercy on me, a sinner") in order to attain union with God.

insight In Buddhism, the understanding of reality; wisdom derived from the practice of concentration (*samadhi*) that leads a seeker to enlightenment or liberation.

jhana (P.) "Meditative absorption." A deep state of concentration in which the mind is single-pointedly focused on the object of meditation.

kaihogyo (J.) Literally, "the practice of circumambulating the mountain." The ascetic practice of walking/running along a set course on Mount Hiei while chanting and stopping to pray at various shrines along the route.

ki (J.) Vital force or energy inherent in any living being; the term translates literally to "air" and more generally to "life force" or "energy flow."

koan (J.) "Public case" or "precedent." Originally a legal term, it now refers to the exchanges culled from historical sources and recorded sayings of the ancient Zen masters. Zen students sit with these koans during meditation, and the intense level of doubt that results is meant to lead them to insight in the form of a sudden breakthrough.

liberation *See* enlightenment.

liturgy Communal worship; the forms that constitute a response to the sacred through the act of praise, thanksgiving, or repentance.

lüng-gom-pa (T.) Spiritual practitioners who focus single-mindedly (*gom*) on the breath through meditative and yogic exercises in order to attain enlightenment.

Mahayana (S.) "Great Vehicle." A school of Buddhism that emerged roughly around the fourth century CE and whose central tenet is the bodhisattva path achieved through three trainings: meditation, ethical conduct, and wisdom.

manas (S.) "Afflicted mentality." The seventh of the eight consciousnesses, which perceives the storehouse consciousness and mistakenly understands it as self.

marathon monks (J.) "Spiritual athletes" who undergo rigorous physical and spiritual training for the purpose of attaining enlightenment; also known as *gyoja*.

mental formations Also "mental objects" and *dharmas* (in the sense of phenomena). In the *Satipatthana Sutta* (The Four Foundations of Mindfulness), mental formations include the five hindrances, the five aggregates, the six sense consciousnesses, the seven factors of enlightenment, and the Four Noble Truths.

Merton, Thomas (1915–1968) An American Trappist monk, theologian, social activist, and author who wrote numerous books about Christian monasticism and spirituality, social justice, and Zen Buddhism, Confucianism, and Taoism.

mind In Buddhism, the sixth sense consciousness, whose object of perception is thought; in certain texts it is synonymous with awareness and on occasion, with truth or reality itself.

mindfulness *See* sati.

Moravec's Paradox The principle that high-level reasoning such as speaking or doing math requires little computation, but low-level sensorimotor skills such as walking are extremely difficult for artificial intelligence to emulate.

Muzhou (780–877 CE) Muzhou Daoming, a ninth-century Chinese Zen master known for his eccentricity; credited with bringing Yunmen to his first experience of enlightenment.

nirvana (S.) Literally "cessation" from the endless cycle of birth and death that leads to suffering.

Noble Eightfold Path The Buddha's Fourth Noble Truth, the path out of suffering; consists of right view, right determination, right speech, right action, right livelihood, right effort, right mindfulness, and right concentration.

oryoki (J.) "The container that holds the right amount to respond to a need." Refers to the large bowl that ordained monastics use for their meals as well as to the formal meal ceremony itself.

overpronation A "rolling in" of the foot during the push-off phase of the gait cycle; often caused by biomechanical problems, it can lead to injuries due to the uneven distribution of weight on the foot, ankle, and knee.

pranayama (S.) "Restraint of breath"; a term used to include a range of practices of breath control. During the Buddha's six years of asceticism, he practiced *pranayama* as a form of self-mortification.

pronation Natural movement of the foot that takes place during walking or running.

realization *See* enlightenment.

relative The physical manifestation of the absolute reality of all things; the world of phenomena; *see also* absolute.

right concentration (S.) *samyak samadhi.* The seventh of the eight factors of the Noble Eightfold Path; in Buddhism concentration is understood as the development the four *jhanas* as the precursors to insight and enlightenment.

right effort (S.) *samyak vayamo.* Includes the desire for development of wholesome actions and cessation of unwholesome ones. More broadly, effort that leads to the alleviation of suffering.

right mindfulness (S.) *samyak sati.* Remaining ardent, alert, and mindful, a practitioner focuses on the four foundations of mindfulness (body, feelings, mind, and mental formations). Together with concentration, mindfulness leads to insight.

samadhi (S.) "Concentration," "one-pointedness of mind"; also the development of concentration to such a degree that subject and object merge. *See* absolute samadhi *and* working samadhi.

sangha (P.) "Community"; literally, "that which is struck together well." Refers in Buddhism to male and female monastics as well as male and female laity. Also one of the Three Treasures (Buddha, Dharma, Sangha).

sati (P.) "Mindfulness" or "memory." The ability to keep an object in mind; also the "seeing" factor of meditation.

seiza (J.) "Proper sitting." The formal way of kneeling on the floor in Japan; also refers to the small wooden benches used in a *zendo*, or meditation hall.

self a person's essential being; in Buddhism, the self does not exist independently, apart from other selves.

Sengcan (496–606 CE) Chinese Zen master and author of the "Faith Mind Poem"; referred to as the Third Ancestor of Zen in China.

sesshin (J.) "Gathering the mind" or "touching the heart-mind." A period of silent intensive group meditation done in Zen monasteries.

shunyata (S.) *See* emptiness.

six sense consciousnesses The way in which sentient beings perceive reality through the six senses of sight, hearing, smell, taste, touch, and thought.

So-o (831–918 CE) A Tendai monk who spent years performing ascetic practices on Mount Hiei and is considered the founder of the *kaihogyo* practice.

storehouse consciousness *See* alaya-vijñana.

stupa (S.) "Heap." A hemispherical structure that normally contains the relics of a renowned monk or nun. The ritual of circumambulating *stupas* is a common practice in Buddhist countries.

suchness S. *tathata*; "is-ness" or "things as they are." Refers to the fundamental nature of all things, their inherent perfection simply by virtue of their existence.

supination "Rolling out" of the foot that transfers the body's weight to the outside of the foot and little toe.

Theravada (P.) School of the Elders. The dominant form of Buddhism in Southeast Asia; harkens back to the time of the Buddha and relies heavily on the study of the Pali Canon.

Tilopa (988–1069 CE) An Indian mystic and tantric practitioner known as the teacher of Naropa.

Vajrayana (S.) "Adamantine vehicle." Refers to the esoteric school of Buddhism as well as the third of the three vehicles: Hinayana (more popularly known as Theravada), Mahayana, and Vajrayana. It is known primarily through the teachings of Tibetan and Bhutanese teachers, ancient and modern.

visualization A mental image that creates a representation of the physical world or an imagined phenomenon, or the generation of that image; used in various fields, including psychology, sports, education, and religion.

Vulture Peak Mountain One of the Buddha's most frequented sites and the place where he offered a number of his discourses—including his teachings on the *Heart Sutra* and *Lotus Sutra*.

working *samadhi* Single-pointed concentration that functions in activity. *See* absolute samadhi.

Xinxin Ming (C.) *See* Faith Mind Poem.

Yogachara (S.) "Practice of Yoga." One of the two main schools of Mahayana Buddhism, it emphasizes the teaching of "mind only" in which reality is understood as inseparable from the mind.

Yunmen (864–949 CE) Chinese Zen master and founder of the Yunmen School, one of the Five Schools of Zen in Tang China.

zabuton (J.) Rectangular mat used for *zazen*, seated meditation.

zafu (J.) Round cushion used in conjunction with the *zabuton* for the practice of *zazen*.

zazen (J.) Form of seated meditation whose purpose is seeing into one's true nature.

Zen (J.) S. *dhyana* and C. *Chan.* Mahayana school of Buddhism whose main practice is *zazen*, seated meditation. It emphasizes the direct realization of the nature of things and emptiness of the self.

Zhaozhou (778–897) One of the most important and revered Chinese Zen masters during the Tang dynasty; best known for the koan "Mu."

Sources

Chapter 1: Practice

Nhat Hanh, Thich. *Understanding Our Mind*. Berkeley: Parallax Press, 2002.

Zen Mountain Monastery. "Zazen Instructions" (illustrated). https://zmm.org/teachings-and-training/meditation-instructions.

Chapter 2: Intent

Dogen, Eihei. "Genjokoan." In *Zen Mountain Monastery Liturgy Book*. Mount Tremper, NY: Dharma Communications Press, 1998.

Murakami, Haruki. *What I Talk about When I Talk about Running: A Memoir*. New York: Alfred A. Knopf, 2007.

Chapter 3: Commitment

Aristotle. *Metaphysics*. Translated by W. D. Ross. The Internet Classics Archive, http://classics.mit.edu/Aristotle/metaphysics.5.v.html.

Bhikkhu Bodhi, trans. "The Guardians of the World." *Access to Insight* (BCBS Edition), June 5, 2010. https://www.accesstoinsight.org/lib/authors/bodhi/bps-essay_23.html.

Ireland, John D., trans. "Tittha Sutta: Sectarians (1)." *Access to Insight* (BCBS Edition), September 3, 2012. www.accesstoinsight.org/tipitaka/kn/ud/ud.6.04.irel.html.

Kant, Immanuel. *Critique of Pure Reason.* Translated and edited by Paul Guyer and Allen W. Wood. New York: Cambridge University Press, 1998.

Levy, Ariel. "Breaking the Waves." *The New Yorker*, February 10, 2014.

Loori, John Daido. "Dongshan's 'Each Stitch.'" In *The True Dharma Eye: Zen Master Dogen's Three Hundred Koans.* Translated with Kazuaki Tanahashi. Boulder: Shambhala Publications, 2009.

Soma Thera. "The Way of Mindfulness: The Satipatthana Sutta and Its Commentary." *Access to Insight* (BCBS Edition), November 30, 2013. www.accesstoinsight.org/lib/authors/soma/wayof.html.

Tharp, Twyla. *The Creative Habit: Learn It and Use It for Life.* New York: Simon and Schuster, 2006.

Chapter 4: Discipline

Muir, John. *The Wilderness World of John Muir: A Selection from His Collected Work.* Edited by Edwin Way Teale. Boston: Mariner Books, 2001.

Nhat Hanh, Thich. *Understanding Our Mind.* Berkeley: Parallax Press, 2002.

———. "The Five Remembrances." In *Chanting from the Heart: Buddhist Ceremonies and Daily Practices.* Berkeley: Parallax Press, 2006.

Shantideva. *The Way of the Bodhisattva.* Translated by Padmakara Translation Group. Boulder: Shambhala Publications, 2006.

Shibayama, Zenkei. "Sen-jo and Her Soul." In *Gateless Barrier: Zen Comments on the Mumonkan.* Boulder: Shambhala Publications, 2000.

Thanissaro Bikkhu, trans. "Upajjhatthana Sutta: Subjects for Contemplation." *Access to Insight* (BCBS Edition), November 30, 2013. www.accesstoinsight.org/tipitaka/an/an05/an05.057.than.html.

Chapter 5: Body

Avila, Saint Teresa of. *Interior Castle*. London: Burns & Oates, 2002.

Bhikkhu Bodhi, trans. *In the Buddha's Words: An Anthology of Discourses from the Pali Cannon*. Somerville, MA: Wisdom Publications, 2005.

Clancy, Kelly. "A Computer to Rival the Brain." *The New Yorker*, February 15, 2017.

Dreyer, Danny. *Chi Running: A Revolutionary Approach to Effortless, Injury-Free Running*. New York: Fireside Books, 2009.

Noakes, Tim. *Lore of Running*. 4th ed. Cape Town, South Africa: Oxford University Press Southern Africa, 2001.

Chapter 6: Effort

Dreyer, Danny. *Chi Running: A Revolutionary Approach to Effortless, Injury-Free Running*. New York: Fireside Books, 2009.

Frazer, Charles. *Cold Mountain*. New York: Grove Press, 1997.

"Right Effort: *Samma Vayamo*." Edited by Access to Insight. *Access to Insight* (BCBS Edition), November 30, 2013. www.accesstoinsight.org/ptf/dhamma/sacca/sacca4/samma-vayamo/index.html.

Thanissaro Bikkhu, trans. "Sona Sutta: About Sona." *Access to Insight* (BCBS Edition), November 30, 2013. www.accesstoinsight.org/tipitaka/an/an06/an06.055.than.html.

Chapter 7: Breath

Bhikkhu Bodhi, trans. *In the Buddha's Words: An Anthology of Discourses from the Pali Cannon*. Somerville: Wisdom Publications, 2005.

Bhikkhu Bodhi and Bhikkhu Ñanamoli, trans. "Satipatthana Sutta." In *The Middle Length Discourses of the Buddha:*

A Translation of the Majjhima Nikaya. Somerville, MA: Wisdom Publications, 2015.

Fronsdal, Gil, trans. "The Discourse on the Applications of Mindfulness: Satipatthana Sutta." www.insightmeditationcenter.org/articles/satipatthanasutta.pdf.

Shankman, Richard. *The Experience of Samadhi: An In-depth Exploration of Buddhist Meditation*. Boulder: Shambhala Publications, 2008.

Shibayama, Zenkei. *Gateless Barrier: Zen Comments on the Mumonkan*. Boulder: Shambhala Publications, 2000.

Thanissaro Bikkhu, trans. "Sedaka Sutta: At Sedaka." *Access to Insight* (BCBS Edition), November 30, 2013. www.accesstoinsight.org/tipitaka/sn/sn47/sn47.019.than.html.

Chapter 8: Mind

Acharya Dhammapala. *A Treatise on the Paramis*. Translated by Bikkhu Bodhi. Kandy, Sri Lanka: Buddhist Publication Society, 1996. https://www.accesstoinsight.org/lib/authors/bodhi/wheel409.pdf.

Bhikkhu Bodhi, trans. *In the Buddha's Words: An Anthology of Discourses from the Pali Cannon*. Somerville, MA: Wisdom Publications, 2005.

Buddhaghosa. *Visuddhimagga*. Translated by Bikkhu Ñanamoli. Kandy, Sri Lanka: Buddhist Publication Society, 2011.

Buswell, Jr., Robert E., and Donald S. Lopez, Jr. *The Princeton Dictionary of Buddhism*. Princeton, NJ: Princeton University Press, 2014.

Csikszentmihalyi, Mihaly. *Flow: The Psychology of Optimal Experience*. New York: Harper Perennial, 1990.

Dillard, Annie. *Pilgrim at Tinker Creek*. New York: Harper Perennial, 1974.

Nhat Hanh, Thich. *Understanding Our Mind*. Berkeley: Parallax Press, 2002.

Roethke, Theodore. "The Waking." In *The Collected Poems of Theodore Roethke*. New York: Anchor Books, 1975.

Schmidt, Amy. *Dipa Ma: The Legacy of a Buddhist Master*. New York: BlueBridge, 2005.

Chapter 9: Pain

Ferguson, Andy. *Zen's Chinese Heritage: The Masters and Their Teachings*. Somerville, MA: Wisdom Publications, 2011.

Kabat-Zinn, Jon. *Mindfulness Meditation for Pain Relief: Guided Practices for Reclaiming Your Body and Mind*. Audio. Boulder: Sounds True, 2010.

Nyanaponika Thera, trans. *Sallatha Sutta: The Dart* (SN 36.6). Kandy, Sri Lanka: Buddhist Publication Society, 1983.

Chapter 10: Creation

Chah, Ajahn. "Clarity of Insight." 1979. www.ajahnchah.org/book/ Clarity_Insight1.php.

Dreyer, Danny. *Chi Running: A Revolutionary Approach to Effortless, Injury-Free Running*. New York: Fireside Books, 2009.

Grierson, Bruce. "What If Age Is Nothing but a Mind-Set?" *The New York Times Magazine*, October 22, 2014.

Khyentse Rinpoche, Dilgo. *Heart Treasure of the Enlightened Ones: The Practice of View, Meditation, and Action*. Translated by Padmakara Translation Group. Boulder: Shambhala Publications, 1992.

Khyentse Rinpoche, Dzongsar. "Pure, Clear, and Vibrant." *Lion's Roar* (May 9, 2016). www.lionsroar.com/pure-clear-and-vibrant/.

"Running as Spiritual Practice." *On Being* [radio program]. Hosted by Krista Tippett. Produced by On Being Studios. August 16, 2016.

Stevens, Wallace. "The Well Dressed Man with a Beard." In *Wallace Stevens: Collected Poetry and Prose*. New York: Library of America, 1997.

Chapter 11: Stillness

Bryanchaninov, Ignatius. *On the Prayer of Jesus: The Classic Guide to the Practice of Unceasing Prayer Found in* The Way of a Pilgrim. Boston: New Seeds Books, 2006.

Eckhart, Meister. *Selected Writings*. Translated by Oliver Davies. New York: Penguin Books, 1994.

Loori, John Daido. "Zhaozhou's Cypress Tree." In *The True Dharma Eye: Zen Master Dogen's Three Hundred Koans*. Translated with Kazuaki Tanahashi. Boulder: Shambhala Publications, 2009.

Merton, Thomas. *Cistercian Life*. Collegeville, MA: Cistercian Book Service, 1974.

Sengcan, Jianzhi. "Faith Mind Poem." In *Zen Mountain Monastery Liturgy Manual*. Mount Tremper, NY: Dharma Communications Press, 1998.

Woodward, F. L., trans. "Adanta Suttas: Untamed." *Access to Insight* (BCBS Edition), November 30, 2013. http://www.accesstoinsight.org/tipitaka/an/an01/an01.031-040x.wood.html.

Chapter 12: Movement

David-Néel, Alexandra. *Magic and Mystery in Tibet*. Escondido, CA: The Book Tree, 2000.

Govinda, Lama Anagarika. *The Way of the White Clouds*. New York: The Overlook Press, 2005.

Stevens, John. *The Marathon Monks of Mount Hiei*. Brattleboro, VT: Echo Point Books and Media, 2013.

Chapter 13: Silence

Dogen, Eihei. "Fukanzazengi: Universal Recommendations for Zazen." Translated by Norman Waddell and Abe Masao. In

The Art of Just Sitting: Essential Writings on the Zen Practice of Shikantaza, edited by John Daido Loori. Somerville, MA: Wisdom Publications, 2004.

Shibayama, Zenkei. "Well-Known Ryutan." In *Gateless Barrier: Zen Comments on the Mumonkan*. Boulder: Shambhala Publications, 2000.

Thanissaro Bhikkhu, trans. "Kolita Sutta: Kolita." *Access to Insight* (BCBS Edition), February 7, 2012.

Thrangu Rinpoche, Khenchen. *Essentials of Mahamudra: Looking Directly at the Mind*. Somerville, MA: Wisdom Publications, 2004.

Chapter 14: Credo

Allison, Jay, and Dan Gediman, eds. *This I Believe: The Personal Philosophies of Remarkable Men and Women*. New York: Henry Holt and Company, 2007.

About the Author

Vanessa Zuisei Goddard is a writer and Zen teacher based in New York City. For the last ten years, Zuisei has been leading retreats and workshops to teach running as a form of moving meditation and as a tool to increase mindfulness, awareness, and presence. Find her online at vanessazuiseigoddard.org.